REVIEWS

A fascinating piece of work on the relationship between body, mind, art and healing, Jill Hayes has made an important contribution to the field of somatics, movement and expressive arts therapy. What gives her writing a particularly vivid relevancy is that it is grounded in her own living experience as a practicioner. She has conveyed something of the philosophy, theory and aesthetic experience of embodiment and creativity that is often difficult to capture in words.

Daria Halprin
Gestalt therapist and expressive arts therapist, writer, and educator. Her publications include *The Expressive Body in Life, Art and Therapy.*

I place this book high on my list of the best written about movement and bodily expression in therapy. I am smitten by the intelligence and clarity of the writing, the quality of the scholarship, and the creative precision of the author's descriptions of her work with others. Nothing can compare with a focus on the embodied image when it comes to making the case for the necessity of the arts in therapy and this book goes even further with its integration of all the arts, spirit, imagination, and depth psychology. The brilliance of this book by Jill Hayes bodes well for the future of the expressive arts therapies worldwide.

Shaun McNiff
Dean and Professor, Lesley University, Cambridge, Massachusetts. Past President of the American Art Therapy Association and author of *Art Heals: How Creativity Cures the Soul, Art as Medicine, Trust the Process* and *Creating with Others.*

I loved reading this beautifully written, sensitive and perceptive work about the history, development and integrative nature of inner-directed dance. Through symbolic narrative, psychological insight, poetic metaphor, research and more, Jill Hayes invites the reader into the dancer's multi-sensory world, giving special attention to practices of embodiment and imagination. *Performing the Dreams of Your Body* is not about dance as a form of entertainment; rather it is about dance as a way to experience, express, communicate and explore the passions and mysteries of the human soul. If you are interested in embodied imagination, emotion, creativity and compassion, don't miss this book!

Joan Chodorow PhD
Dance therapist, analyst member, C. G. Jung Institute of San Fransisco. Author of *Dance Therapy and Depth Psychology:The Moving Imagination*, editor of *Jung on Active Imagination* and author of *Active Imaginiation: Healing from Within.*

Fear is one of the great inhibitors to learning; fear of inadequacy, of not measuring up to the standards of our peers. From early on in our lives we are told we are not good enough, and we store the hurt in our bodies, hiding it away from others.

Jill Hayes embarks on a quest to honour individuality and find a healing path that releases energy so that it can flow between mind, body and spirit. Though the brain is prioritised in western society, it cannot function without the physical body, and if the body is freed from the negative patterns, life can become so much more agreeable. Listen to the body and its innate wisdom: there are so many intelligences to be discovered.

Jill writes from personal experience and discussions with students over many years. She introduces techniques that help to build self-belief and shed trauma and, as knowledge is gained about the discipline of movement therapy, so tensions of rigid learning can be released and the internal dynamics of the body's own natural rhythms can begin to be understood. Then the body discovers an 'energy beyond conscious awareness' and releases the creativity that is a part of our humanness.

This is a book that promotes self-knowledge and helps to dispense with self-doubt. It is authoritative and yet accessible, with an approach that is gentle but nonetheless powerful. Dance practitioners will be enriched by the knowledge she has to impart.

Dr Ann Nugent

Senior Lecturer in Dance at the University of Chichester. Internationally acclaimed dance writer and teacher. Former editior of *Dance Now* and *Dance Theatre Journal*.

This is a truly blessed work. The title gives us an indication of the depth of its content. The book gives us a glimpse of the body as incarnation of soul impregnated with spirit. In her attempt to put into verbal language the amazing embodied experiences and performances she has witnessed, Jill has managed to integrate the poet with the researcher, the receptive with the proactive, the feminine with the masculine.

Professor Helen Payne

Professor in Counselling and Psychotherapy, University of Hertfordshire. Dance movement therapist and psychotherapist. Editor-in-Chief of the international journal *Body, Movement and Dance in Psychotherapy* and author of several books including: *Dance Movement Therapy, Theory, Practice and Research*.

Performing the Dreams of Your Body

Plays of Animation and Compassion

To dear Eva,
Our work together
has brought me so much
joy in this
crazy old
world!

Lots of
love,
Jill
x

Performing the Dreams
of Your Body

Plays of
Animation and Compassion

Jill Hayes

Jill Hayes

26.

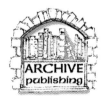

ARCHIVE
publishing

CHICHESTER ENGLAND

MMVII

viii

First published in Great Britain by

ARCHIVE PUBLISHING
Chichester, England.

Designed for Archive Publishing by Ian Thorp

A CIP Record for this book is available from
the British Cataloguing in Publication data office

ISBN 978-1-906289-01-0 Hardback
ISBN 978-1-906289-00-3 Paperback

Front cover image: 'Renaissance Symposium: enquiry into the soul'
Carol Lloyd, November, 2006

Photograph of Jill Hayes: Graham Sherlock

Printed and bound in England by
LIGHTNING SOURCE

DEDICATION

To my sister Marie-Therese Arnoux.

Body and Soul

My soul is patiently waiting for a vessel
Longing to be contained,
Longing to be carried by my body,
For my body is the vessel through which
My soul can be and unfold.
Without it, my soul is like a seed
Which has nowhere to grow

Claudine McTaggart, 2007
(an extract from the poem)

ACKNOWLEDGEMENTS

I want to thank you Moira Dadd, Kelly Holmes, Wynona Kaspar, Tracie Masterman, Catherine McLelland, Merle, Caroline Ohlson, Caroline Pearce-Higgins, Amie Powlesland, Sarah Reed and Ana Rezende-Miggin for giving your stories to this book. Without these stories there would be no book!

I also want to thank all the people who took part in the research through participation in experiential work and questionnaire response. It is your voices which enliven the analysis.

Thank you to all my colleagues and friends for inspiration, in particular to Dr Marie Angelo whose vision of 'imaginatio enquiry' has given me confidence and purpose, and to Professor Valerie Briginshaw who created the space for the book to be written.

Finally, I want to thank my family: my father Thomas Hayes and my mother Dyllys Hayes, my husband Paul Wilson, and our sons Finny, Lawrie, Owain and Theo, whose love brings me joy. For joy, the child of love, writes these pages.

Although every effort has been made to gain permission for all the quotations, some sources remain unlocatable at the time of going to press. We wish to acknowledge and thank the sources of all quotations that appear and in particular:

Central Europe Gallery and Publishing House, Prague - *Transmutation of the Senses* - Svankmajer.
City Lights Publishing - *Isadora Speaks* - Rosemont.
Dallas Institute of Humanities and Culture - *Fragments of a Poetics of Fire* - Bachelard.
Inner City Books - *Jung and Yoga* - Harris.
Norton - *The Neuroscience of Psychotherapy* - Cozolino.
Princetown University Press - *Collected Works* - Jung.
Princeton Book Co - *The Modern Dance* - Martin.
Routledge - *Modern Man in Search of a Soul* - Jung.
Shambhala Publications - *Art Heals* - McNiff.
            - Art as Medicine - McNiff.
            - *Knowing Woman* - Claremont de Castillejo.

All sources appear in full in the References.

CONTENTS

FOREWORD

Professor Helen Payne

This is a truly blessed work. The title of this book – *Performing the Dreams of your Body: Plays of Animation and Compassion* – gives us an indication of the depth of its content. This book shows us a glimpse of body as incarnation of soul impregnated with sprit. A 'suffering with' is presented, from which new community is co-created and compassion experienced by both witness and mover.

Jill says the book wrote itself; and my experience on reading it was that it read itself. The reading required no effort on my part. I feel grateful for that lightness. In the stream of ideas presented, fed by the poems and voices of participants, I experienced a gentle touch. My imagination was stimulated by each performance as it played out human conflicts in a symbolic process of expression and containment.

I am privileged to have been a witness to Jill's journey through her doctoral research since 1997. When we first met she was keen to inquire into the nature of dance movement therapy (DMT) with dance students. Since my primary interest has always been researching clients' perceptions of the therapeutic process, I immediately felt an attunement with her ideas. I noticed Jill had qualities of warmth and rigour as her elegiac language flowed freely over me. Since that first meeting I have witnessed her surmount many obstacles on her pathway towards the successful dawn of her doctorate, as well as birthing two more children!

At the university graduation ceremony in the sacred space of St Alban's Abbey I had the honour of presenting her, which I undertook with reverence. At that time we briefly spoke of her new journey, the writing of this book. I felt then, as now, immensely joyful that the wonderful work which she had spent so long refining and painstakingly sweating over would speak to a wider audience. At all times Jill has sought to place the voices of the participants in the forefront of her writing. I am struck by how fundamental these voices are in this book.

Reading her work again, I can see how she has built on her previous findings. Another, further integration is evident. The healing she spoke of for her dance students in her thesis has now included spirit in a much more central place. As I read I am moved to reflect on my own path and the importance of finding spirit within myself through my own mindful, expressive movement and witnessing experiences in Authentic Movement.

This book is a reflective account of journeys into the unknown, using organically evolved movement plays. The prime focus is the nature of the transpersonal in Jill's rich contribution to the field of dance and dance movement therapy (DMT). Transcendence is associated with the heights of spirit, in contrast to the descent to soul. Her writing emphasises the unity of spirit with soul and underpins the connections between moving and imagination. It is both poetic and scholarly, not easy to achieve in one volume. Jill draws her inspiration from the participants' descriptive accounts of their plays: these plays 'are unique and various, but contain threads of commonality, in the interplay between polarities of motion, emotion and imagery', she writes (p. xviii), adding that embodied imagination heightens awareness of opposites to bring balance. She reminds us that both psyche and matter are required for transformation. She suggests we follow Jung's advice: we need to dive into the chaos and begin to separate out the opposites, to participate in the process of consciousness (p. 6).

The term 'play' is chosen by Jill because of its symbolic quality. It is linked with human nature, and mirrors our internal world. She uses the term 'anima' not as soul, as does Jung, but to describe 'receptive and prospective energies in a dance of energy or spirit' (p. xix). The calling for the book came from the energy taken in and through the body. That which needs to incarnate becomes matter in the embodied imagination. The book's contention is that identification with, and holding of, emotions may happen through our dreaming body and our imagination. We can suffer with ourselves and with the other as witness, identifying through the body with the play of another; and with this Jill makes a plea for a return to what she calls the 'bodyspirit' (p. 2).

In this book, I see a leap of insight, from the creative process of academic research into a new place of integration rooted in bodyspirit. This is embodied research, transpersonal research even. Perhaps bodyspirit is that place that lies between the body and BodySoul (a term used by Marion Woodman in her BodySoul Rhythm work). The body lives its truth and moves spirit to find a new wholeness as bodyspirit. I can imagine a crystal with three faces: 'body – BodySoul – bodyspirit'.

The heart of this book is the embodied human being. Life itself is mirrored in our journey through the pages. The deep connection which is made with body, nature and the rhythms of our earth is profoundly humbling. Arising out of this deep connection with that powerful, awesome place – earth, body, matter – come animation, spirit, love and compassion in the form of poems, creative reflections and inspired writing. My imagination was indeed stirred to roam freely in and out of the scenes co-created by Jill and the voices of her participants. These performances are enthralling. The framework Jill uses to capture their communication within community speaks to the heart and soul within me. I do feel moved to move! We are designed to move and it is in the body, spontaneously moving with imagination, feeling and community, that the direct experience of the self, and of life itself, can be profoundly felt.

It is refreshing to find participants so engaged with the research process that they feel a desire to be seen by the collective. And so their own names appear in the text: Moira with her act of courage; Caroline finding her voice; Wynona and her seed for growth; Ana's spirit manifested in eternal rhythm; Catherine and her bird of fire; Merle's sea animal and the four performers – Kelly, Tracie, Amie and Sarah – in 'Stone'. I can clearly see each one of them, and I can see spirit unfolding on the pages of this book. I am the one for whom the words therein resonate deeply. The receiving and channelling through the body of anima, energy and spirit are seen as fundamental to the creative process; this process applies equally to life and to art.

In her attempt to put into words the amazing embodied experiences and performances she has witnessed, Jill has managed to integrate the poet with the researcher, the receptive with the proactive, the feminine with the masculine. Authentic Movement practice is an aspect of DMT entirely suited to transpersonal or psychospiritual work. It is a fundamental ingredient of psychotherapy. Healing, it could be argued, cannot take place without a corresponding change in the transpersonal, through embodied spirit. The ideas Jill contributes to transpersonal dance movement form another useful framework for the evolving nature of DMT theory, research and practice. And including bodyspirit in a truly holistic approach to dance training, education and practice will surely invite compassionate performers and audiences to the shrine of spirit in community.

There is a suggestion that the heightened awareness of the perceptual and expressive body is also a tool in the verbal therapeutic relationship. It is made clear towards the end of the book that transpersonal dance movement can be usefully employed in the continuing professional development of counsellors and psychotherapists, which I can fully endorse since I engage with this in my own practice.

I sincerely recommend this book to those involved in dance movement therapy, visual art, dance and spiritual practices of any kind. It is a gem to treasure. I hope it will be read by practitioner, client and trainer both present and future. It will surely develop a depth of understanding of the processes involved when embodiment becomes the seed and flower of that which is heartfelt.

When Jill asked me to write the Foreword to her book I felt nervous about agreeing, fearing that I would not do justice to the work. However, I have been surprised that, as reading it was effortless, so writing this reflection on its content has had a quality of flow and simplicity. I hope my words have done full justice to the book. It has been a pleasure for me to read it and write about it. I hope it gives you, dear reader, as much pleasure.

Thank you Jill, and all your participants, for this beautiful artefact of the spirit of embodiment.

Professor Helen Payne
University of Hertfordshire
Hatfield, England.
May 2006

PROLOGUE

Performing the dreams of your body can be transformative. When you read these plays of animation and compassion, you will see how openness to body and imagination through transpersonal dance movement practice has helped dancers, visual artists and therapists to gain a stronger sense of personal history, personal power and transpersonal connection. I use the term 'transpersonal' broadly, to mean 'beyond the personal'. It encompasses depth connection with other people (inter-subjectivity) and with the natural world of living organisms, and it embraces the concept of a vital energy or spirit permeating the earth and cosmos.

I describe the movement-based work of this book as transpersonal dance movement practice: an approach to dance and movement which is transpersonal, and which draws on several disciplines and practices, acknowledged in Part 1. This work is not therefore a single established form; it has been influenced by a wide range of transpersonal and transformative dance movement practices, all of which have absolute respect for the experience of body, soul and spirit. Body is defined as the unique physical form of the individual, soul as the unique inner experience of the individual coloured by emotion, intuition and creativity[1] and spirit as transpersonal energy animating the cosmos. Soul is sometimes used interchangeably with psyche, and whilst I refer to an inner creativity, I suggest connection with an eternal soul or spirit, still there when our human ego and consciousness have disappeared.[2]

One of the most influential transpersonal dance movement practices in the work here described is Authentic Movement, which is capitalised to indicate a particular discipline of practice, developed by Mary Starks Whitehouse as 'movement-in-depth' in the mid-twentieth century. Sometimes I use the word 'authentic' without capitals to indicate organic movement arising in the body from an 'inner impulse'.[3]

---

1   Moore, 1992.
2   Hillman, 1975, p. xvi.
3   Whitehouse, 1958a, 1958b, 1978, 1979.

The experience of embodiment with imagination has made a significant impact upon the lives and work of the people represented in this book. These people are either students or professionals in the fields of dance, visual art or psychotherapy. Transpersonal dance movement practice has altered how they are and how they approach their work. The plays may therefore be offered in support of the suggestion that learning from body and imagination through transpersonal dance movement practice may be applied to dance, visual art and psychotherapy training and continuing professional development.

You will witness both individual and group dances of emotion and imagination, and you will be shown the internal processes of the students, as they have awakened to body messages and communicated felt-experience through body metaphor. Despite their different disciplines, all students have shared an interest in letting their bodies receive and express their emotions and their imagination. They have believed that the creative relationship between body, emotion and imagination has something to offer; that befriending embodied emotions and images can bring inspiration, reconciliation and guidance.

The dances are unique and various, but contain threads of commonality, in the interplay between polarities of motion, emotion and imagery. This commonality seems to suggest that embodied emotion and imagination can heighten awareness of opposites and can bring balance.

The term 'play' is chosen to define the dance processes and performances because of its dual meaning. The little child immersed in creative play moves fluidly with images as they enter the mind. In authentic movement we find again that liquid state of creative play, unafraid to embody imagination. Unimpeded by external aesthetic or moral judgement we are able to allow the movements, images and feelings to develop as they arise.

The play as performance may be created as a reflection of human experience or as Shakespeare suggests in Hamlet, Act III, Scene II:

> The purpose of playing ... is, to hold, as 'twere,
> the mirror up to nature.[4]

Perhaps therefore the play may be perceived as a revelation of nature in us. 'Nature' may be defined as something living, energetic, animated; that which grows and moves. The play helps us to see what is alive, growing and moving in us. It becomes a container for organic processes.

I use the term 'animation' to describe the plays. The verb 'to animate' comes from the Latin 'animare', which means 'to endue with life' and 'anima', translated as 'life' and 'breath'. Spirit, from the Latin 'spiritus', is also translated as 'breath'.[5] These derivations weave anima, spirit and breath into one concept. Anima, spirit and breath are often perceived as a unity in transpersonal dance movement practice, and our breath becomes a focus in our intention to connect with anima or spirit. It is through the energetic experience of breath that we feel enlivened by anima or spirit.

Jung refers to 'anima' as a feminine potential, differentiating this from 'animus', a masculine potential. My reference to 'anima' is different. It adheres to the Latin definition of 'anima' as life and breath, and I wish through my use of 'anima' to indicate both receptive and prospective energies as partners in a dance of anima or spirit.

The definition of anima or spirit as it is used in this book is close to the Chinese concept of 'ch'i': a vital, eternal energy permeating earth and cosmos. In transpersonal dance movement practice I experience a vital energy taken in through my breath, passing through and enlivening my body. I feel this energy through all the surfaces of my body, as I dance on the earth, as I move in the air. The vibration of energy passes into me from outside and fills me with life. I do not suggest divinity in my definition of energy, but I do speak of an eternal process, which is wild, grand and terrible.

---

4   Shakespeare [1564-1616], 1968.
5   Skeat, 1978, p. 508.

Thus, anima, spirit and energy are used here synonymously to describe an invisible eternal process which may be physically perceived and imaginatively embodied to tell our human story. This invisible process may be compared and contrasted with Hillman's concept of soul as a 'self-sustaining and imagining substrate'.[6] I am suggesting that the 'self-sustaining substrate' is perceived energetically first then evolves into image. Woodman[7] likens archetypal forms to iron filings pulled by a magnet into shapes from underneath a paper. In the same way eternal process may swirl inside us and take form. We sense transpersonal energy in our own bodies, in other people, in animals and in the natural world. We transform and communicate this energy through our imaginative bodies.[8]

When we feel lost and cannot move spontaneously, we can always return to the rhythm of the breath, which allows the potential patterns of the body to unfold. It is the rhythm of the breath which feeds our bodies, and facilitates the emergence of movement and counter-movement. As we breathe out, we curl inwards and close, then breathing in we uncurl outwards and open. Breathing out and in, we find that we mirror patterns in the plant and animal world and feel in our bodies our connection to the earth.

I suggest that transpersonal energy is present in the passion of the plays in this book and appears in many different images. Some images are feminine (e.g. mother), or have become feminised in some cultures (e.g. earth, sea); some have become masculinised (e.g. phoenix, sun, fire); yet here they are all offered as expressions of eternal energy transformed by soul.

Most of the images have a cultural history. It was not the intention of the movement work, nor the intention of this book, to explore in depth historical and cultural precedents. The work was organic[9] and phenomenological[10]: images were tended as they surfaced in our bodies so that we became conscious of

---

6   Hillman, 1975, p. xvi.
7   Woodman, 1993, p. 151.
8   Chodorow, 1991.
9   Clements, Ettling, Jenett, Shields, 1998.
10   Valle, Mohs, 1998.

their potential in the present moment. By experiencing and dwelling with the images which presented themselves through embodied imagination, we sought to find out their significance for the protagonist and for the performance community. We did not seek to explain the source of energy but to explore the experience of energy in body, emotions and imagination, within and between people.

The phenomenology of movement tells us about ourselves as unique individuals and also about ourselves as human beings; it connects us to others. I am suggesting that subjectivity may be the basis of archetypal and mythic experience: through immersion in the subjective, we transcend the subjective. In dwelling with our own story we move organically through it and beyond it; we are released from it. From a place of physical, emotional and imaginative knowing we are able to reach out to others. Our story becomes myth or archetype, speaking of our humanity.

I use the word 'compassion' to describe the plays. Compassion derives from the Latin 'com' which means 'with' and 'passio' which means suffering. So we suffer or endure with others, when we feel compassion for them. The Latin word 'sufferre' from which suffer derives means 'to undergo' or 'to bear',[11] suggesting a keen ability to be present in the life situation in which we find ourselves. The concept of being present is central to the practice of both humanistic and transpersonal psychotherapy, where the term 'congruence'[12] is chosen to express present experience and awareness of physical, emotional and mental states. Suffering then is about receptivity to the immediate experience of body and mind; a turning towards life. Compassion is a willingness to share the physical, emotional and mental state of others without judgement and with a sense of equality.

Jungian/existential analyst and writer Linda Leonard[13] writes of the importance of learning to bear/hold the emotional pain of existence (to suffer), in order to feel alive and in relationship with

---

11   Skeat, 1978, p. 528.

12   Rogers, 1957; Wyatt, 2001.

13   Linda Leonard, 1989.

others. This book's contention is that the identification with and holding of emotions may happen through our body and through our imagination.[14] Despite armouring,[15] I suggest that our bodies always retain a core responsiveness: they can and do respond to life with a spontaneity which analytic thought will often try to quell and re-represent. Therefore it is to our bodies that we must turn if we want to bear our truth. Imagination helps us in this intention, for imagination can hold physical and emotional truth through the forms it creates.[16]   Compassionate performance offers a sensitive, receptive public forum to assist in the bearing of emotions.

In the plays of this book the protagonists learn to bear their truth by working with their bodies and their imaginations. This gives rise to compassion. This compassion is twofold, for it is a *suffering with ourselves* as we breathe life into our suffering through creative movement, as it is the *suffering with the other* as we witness and identify through our bodies with the play of another. The 'holding circle'[17] of the group is a visual image for a united   compassionate   presence,   which   launches   the protagonists in their venture to bear or suffer their truth.

Clearly the plays in this book can be interpreted from different heuristics. For example, embodied images may be worked with psychodynamically,   explained   as   repressed   desires,   sub-personalities or complexes finding their way to consciousness through sublimation. But ego-oriented theories do not match the experience of the players. Human fragility and permeability is often conceptualised as pathology in these frameworks, whereas transpersonal frameworks refer to mystery, beauty, destruction, creation, soul and spirit. Ego-oriented theories do not discuss the concept of energy beyond the individual, nor do they examine the existential and archetypal substance of our humanity. A transpersonal framework is favoured because it reflects the spiritual, existential and archetypal experience of the players.

---

14   Chodorow, 1991; Gendlin, 1981; Halprin, 2003.
15   Reich, 1933.
16   Cox and Theilgaard, 1987.
17   Chapter 2, Section 2.5

When we focus on body-felt experience we can alter our perception and our conceptualisation of ourselves in the world. Embodiment helps us to find a raw energy, stark, potent and creative, untamed by self-protecting and self-confining judgement and categorisation. My experience is that when we let ourselves be open to the presence of energy lying dormant inside us, we wake up to untapped potential. Such potential can feed our creative life; it offers rhythm and pattern to our imagination.

As a dance movement therapist and Authentic Movement practitioner I have witnessed energy awakening in the body. When a person begins to move with faith in the body (begins to 'be moved'[18]), emotion and metaphor also begin emerge spontaneously. When this happens, something changes. The relationship to self, to others and to the world is different, because this process takes us to spirit. Spirit fills the soul, the inner space, and gives energy to the heart of human experience. With spirit we can experience the human passions which move, bewilder, frighten and inspire us, and we can feel the thunder-roll of destiny: our potential existence.

Transpersonal dance movement practice may be seen as defiance against rigid structures, enclosing and defining who we are in materialistic, society-bound terms. Befriending our body, our emotions and our imagination reawakens an inner yearning for self-care, self-expression and transcendence. Transpersonal dance movement practice both acknowledges and feeds our 'hunger' to belong to something bigger than a separate human identity.[19]

It has been a pleasure and an honour to devote my attention to the embodied stories of my students. First in witnessing them I have been physically and emotionally moved and inspired. Then in reflecting upon them over these months of writing, I have felt again the songs and the dances, and I realise that I am not alone, that I am part of a great dance of humanity and

---

18   Whitehouse, 1958a, 1958b, 1972, 1978, 1979.
19   O'Donohue, 1998.

connected to spirit.[20] So I am expanded and enlarged by your processes and performances. I am taken beyond myself. Thank you. To me it seems that the book has almost written itself, carried by the inspiration I have gained from your work.

Part 1: Behind the Scenes shows the thinking and practice behind the book. It gives a rationale for working with the body to experience spirit and describes a spontaneous, interconnected process of motion, emotion and imagination. Chapter 1 begins with a plea for the forgotten body and for a return to a holistic concept of bodyspirit. Comparative definitions of body, mind and spirit from archetypal psychology, neuroscience, transpersonal somatic practice, mysticism and transpersonal dance, help to identify the concepts as used in the book. The choice of these disciplines for comparative theories and ideas is determined by the book's focus on the application of body knowledge to psychotherapy training and dance education. The chapter proposes a fluid relationship between spirit, body, emotion and imagination, and suggests that the body can be both perceiver and imaginative expresser of spirit. Chapter 2 then discusses the processes of embodiment behind the book, with particular reference to the discipline of Authentic Movement. I begin with my movement experience at Tamalpa Institute, co-founded by Anna and Daria Halprin, and subsequently explore movement processes in Authentic Movement, Dharma Art, transpersonal dance and dance movement therapy (DMT). I acknowledge faltering processes of mind and advocate the responsive creation of a safe, egalitarian, bonded community, which becomes the home for compassionate, healing performance. The chapter closes with a reflection on the difficulty of writing about live processes; inevitably the poetic translation is different from the original; something new, but rooted in the original experience, is created. Part 2 (Chapters 3 to 7) gives you the plays of animation and compassion, most of which were originally witnessed as performances in the class community. The themes have been divided into chapters on mother and child, earth, fire, stone and sea animal. Yet the plays are all

---

20   Houston, 1987.

interlinked. They all show how the human story and the stories of the planet are found through the earth of the body, soaring on the wings of imagination. Part 3: Epilogue contains reflections from research and practice, drawing on students' impressions of their processes of embodiment and the repercussions for their life and work. Chapter 8 focuses on undergraduate and postgraduate dancers and visual artists, and Chapter 9 on postgraduate professional psychotherapists. This final part of the book makes some recommendations for inclusion of transpersonal dance movement practice, as illustrated in the book, in the training of dancers, visual artists and psychotherapists. Chapter 10 is a brief farewell to bodyspirit. I hope that you enjoy reading the book and that you will be inspired to move!

INTERLUDE

Before I begin, I want to tell you a story based on Hans Christian Anderson's (1805-1875) original version of 'The Nightingale'. This story honours the unintelligible and un-containable nature of the energy which I am also calling anima or spirit. The metaphor of the nightingale's song is an eloquent representation of the concept of energy, for song is vibration. In 'Performing the Dreams of Your Body' I am telling about the experience of energy, but not suggesting that it is knowable or conceivable to the human mind. I am simply writing about perceived experiences of connection with an animating process. It seems vital to me to resist the ego's desire to take ownership of spirit, and it is a challenge to learn how to observe and be with its presence. This story of 'The Emperor's Nightingale' shows how the temptation to possess and control spirit leads to the temptation of manufacturing spirit. Devotion to spiritless, materialistic beauty estranges the emperor from that which is essential in the nightingale's song. It is only when near to death that he can listen to the song again and appreciate the vast and mysterious nature of spirit.

In writing this book I have wanted to stay true to students' experience of spirit, and not to manufacture beautiful imitations. All contributors have read the representations of their stories and given their permission for them to be published (giving their identity, except in one instance where we chose a fictional name) as accurate reflections of their soulful experience.

The Emperor's Nightingale

Once upon a time there was a Chinese emperor who lived in the most magnificent palace in the world. His gardens, in which the most beautiful flowers bloomed, were enchanted and magical. There was a nightingale, who had made a nest on one of the branches of a flowering tree. The bird's song was so glorious that everyone around stopped working just to listen to it.

When the emperor heard of this, he flew into a rage."Who does this nightingale think he is? He lives in my garden and I have never heard him. Bring him to me and let him sing to me in person!"

A golden twig was placed in front of the emperor and the little grey bird was brought before him. The little bird sang so divinely that tears came to the emperor's eyes. As the tears ran down the old man's cheeks, the song of the nightingale grew sweeter and sweeter. His voice touched everyone's heart and he became a star.

Then one day the emperor received a large parcel containing a mechanical nightingale. It was designed to imitate the real nightingale and was covered with diamonds, rubies and sapphires. It was so beautiful and like the other it sang so well that everyone wanted to hear the two nightingales sing in concert. So they were made to sing together. But the duet sounded quite wrong, because the real nightingale sang from natural inspiration and the other followed its mechanical movement. So the artificial bird was made to sing alone. It was as popular as the real bird and was far more pleasing to the eye, because it sparkled with precious jewels.

It sang the same passage thirty-three times over without becoming in the least bit tired, and so pleased the crowd that they chased the real nightingale away. The real nightingale was banished from the city and the empire, and the artificial bird took the seat of honour on a little lacquered table beside the emperor's bed.

But one evening when the mechanical bird was singing his heart out and the emperor was listening enraptured from his bed, there was a sudden "crack" from inside the bird's body, then a "br-rr-oo-oo". All the gear wheels jammed and the music stopped abruptly. The wonderful mechanism had rusted. The mechanical bird would never sing again.

Five years later the country was plunged into deepest gloom. The Chinese greatly loved their emperor and he had fallen ill, and it was said that he was about to die. The old emperor lay pale and cold in his bed. He found it so hard to breathe, he felt as if people were trampling on his chest. As he opened his eyes he saw Death. It had come to fetch him and he was very frightened at the thought that his last hour had come.

Then suddenly from the window a delightful song was heard. It was the little nightingale from the forest, who sat trilling on a branch. It had learned of the emperor's illness and had come to cheer him up and to bring him hope. The little nightingale sang so beautifully and so sweetly that the emperor's terrible visions of death disappeared. As if by magic, the old man was cured and regained his strength immediately.

"Thank you, thank you, heavenly little bird," he exclaimed. "I once chased you away and yet your singing has chased away the evil spirits. How can I reward you?"

"You have already rewarded me," sang the nightingale. "I brought tears to your eyes the first time I sang. For me, those were diamonds and I shall never forget them. Let me come and visit you whenever I can. I shall sing to you of the joyful and the sad, about good and evil, about all the things you know nothing about, because a little bird flies everywhere and sees everything. Only promise me one thing, do not tell anyone that you have a little bird who tells you everything. Believe me, it is for the best."

And the little nightingale flew away. A moment later the courtiers and servants entered the room to see the dying emperor for the last time. They were astonished when the emperor sat up and wished them a hearty, "Good day!" [21]

---

[21]   Burnford & Barnham, eds., 1997.

Part 1

Behind the Scenes

In this part of the book I want to show you the thinking and practice behind the plays of animation and compassion which you will witness in Part 2. In Chapter 1 I show you my own thinking on bodyspirit and how it is similar to and different from other concepts of body, soul and spirit from archetypal psychology, neuroscience, transpersonal somatic practice, mysticism and transpersonal dance. Ideas from these disciplines were particularly sought because of the book's focus on the application of body knowledge to psychotherapy training and dance education.

I offer a non-hierarchical view of transpersonal energy, manifesting in body, emotions and imagination. I believe that body movement, emotion and imagination are all forms of transpersonal energy, of equal bounty and wonder. I do not suggest that body energy must be refined into 'higher' forms of energy in order to achieve a superior state, but see the dance between energy and form as a continual process of balance between being and creativity, experiencing and reflection, feeling and awareness.

Chapter 2 shows the processes of embodiment behind the practice and plays of the book. I concentrate on my own experience because this has informed my practice, but I embrace other processes of embodiment in dance, which draw upon emotion and imagination in similar ways.

Chapter 1

A philosophy of bodyspirit

There are more things in heaven and earth, Horatio,
Than are dreamt of in your philosophy.[22]

1.1: Spirit is in the body

We are sensate beings in a sensate world, constantly in sensate relationship with the people and the environment surrounding us. It is through our bodies that we make and break contact with our sensate world. In the womb as the body grows and develops we perceive everything around us through our bodies. Our bodies are ourselves in this world; they are the source of our knowledge about ourselves and the world.

What happens to us as we grow older? We often lose identification with our bodies, and we lose respect for our bodies. We focus upon one part of our bodies: the brain, rather than attending to the whole body, as a system in which kinaesthetic, visceral and labyrinthine perception plays an important part. We tend to hold the brain in high regard to the exclusion of its companion body. But the brain needs the rest of the body, just as the rest of the body needs the brain. They work together as a system for experiencing, making sense of and expressing self and the world.

For there can be no connection between us, others and the world, if not through the mediation of the senses. James Hillman,[23] writer, lecturer, analyst, and author of many complex works discussing pluralistic visions of archetypal psychology, remarks that many contemporary western cultures have lost a relationship with beauty, which he equates with the 'sensate

---

22   Hamlet Prince of Denmark, Act I, Scene V, Shakespeare [1564-1616], 1968.
23   James Hillman, 1992.

presence' of the world. I contend that we have lost this because we have lost our relationship with our bodies. O'Donohue,[24] philosopher, poet and mystic, writes of our hunger to belong to a sensate presence in nature. How can we feel this but through our bodies? And feel it we can, when we quieten our thoughts and feel our bodies' energy. In Anam Cara, O'Donohue writes:

> Attunement to the senses ... can warm and heal the atrophied feelings which are the barriers that exile us from our selves and separate us from each other.[25]

When we let go of logical thinking, we let spirit dance inside us, awakening emotion and image, and in being present with this experience we connect with corresponding energetic, emotional and imaginative experience in others and in nature. For this to happen, we must have faith that we (as human entity) will not cease to exist, but rather be enlivened and expanded by the presence of spirit. It is a matter of trusting spirit to repair, nurture and transform us whilst in our human form, rather than fearing that our human identity will be taken away.

It is in the turning inwards with eyes closed that we enhance our sensate experience. We begin to sense the rhythms in the body, focusing on our breath, and our pulse. As we let our breath move us, rhythm becomes pattern and we begin to have a sense of balancing, cyclic movement in the body, such as the perennial dance of extension and contraction, the spine and the body opening and closing, the extension reaching as far as it can then turning into contraction.

Through embodiment of swooping figures of eight, of waves and spirals we can connect to plant forms and to the elements of nature. Or feeling the weight of the body, we sink our hands and knees as four paws into the ground, and push forwards from the pelvis. The loops of the pelvis create a wave through the skeleton and we become the body of a wildcat.

---

24   O'Donohue, 1998.
25   O'Donohue, 1999, p. 85, from Anam Cara by John Donohue, published by Bantam Press. Reprinted by permission of the Random House Group Ltd.

When we experience movement in this way we can feel and imagine ourselves as part of the plant world, the elemental world and the animal world, unfurling outwards and curling inwards, spiralling and swirling forwards, looping, weaving through space. In this way consciousness of our connection to energy in nature is born on the waves of the senses. The authentic movements I make are experienced as reflections of nature.

Rhythm and pattern exist in us and around us, in all movements of destruction and creation on earth. The breaking down and reassembling of matter is in constant flux, in the changing of caterpillar into butterfly or in the dropping and decay of the apple inside the earth. I feel creation and destruction physically inside my body as a woman, in the cycle of menstruation, in the process of gestation and giving birth. The growing of cells and a baby inside me, and now the aging of my body, give me a strong physical sense of being part of a cycle of life and death. Thus the very physical being of my body as well as the organic and imaginative movement of my body bring me into relationship with spirit.

Students describing transformative dance often refer to being moved by energy; the movement makes itself. This is sometimes perceived as thrilling or releasing, and sometimes as bewildering or even frightening. It is a challenge to accept this energy and to let it live inside; it is an act of surrender. When I feel energy awakening and I do not fight against it, I may begin to feel that I am discovering a creative power beyond me and in me.[26] I need to trust in my body to tell the human story of this potential. These moments of accepting and being moved by energy are moments of unity; they are an expression of bodyspirit.

The relationship between body, mind and spirit has been debated so often that this in itself illustrates the tendency to see them as separate entities instead of as a whole.[27] In this book I am defining body as our physical being; mind, psyche and soul

---

[26]   McNiff, 2004; Rogers, 2000.
[27]   Hartley, 2004.

as our creative, intuitive being, or inner space; and spirit as the vital energy which permeates all things on earth and in the cosmos. Emotions are considered as present in both body and soul, igniting movement and imagination.[28] In sensitive and responsive relationship, these aspects of being are seen as potentially capable of transforming one into the other, in fluid cycles. Body, mind and spirit are therefore perceived to be part of a relational system, in which movement, emotion, image and thought are all energetically interconnected.

Jung, founder of archetypal psychology, perceived body, mind and spirit as a whole entity. The physical and spiritual are seen as two aspects of the same thing. He imagined a holistic synthesis between the material, the psychic and the spiritual, and suggested that the challenge for humankind was to experience this unity by being present in body, mind and spirit. He writes:

> Since psyche and matter are contained in one and the same world, and moreover are in continuous contact with one another and ultimately rest on irrepresentable, transcendental factors, it is not only possible but fairly probable, even, that psyche and matter are two different aspects of one and the same thing. [29]

Moving with Jungian theory, I have sought to grow down behind my personality/ mask into my body to connect with spirit. Jung sees the instinctual and physiological as the 'prima materia' to which we must, like the alchemists, return. For it is here that we will experience the chaotic and undifferentiated energy of the 'divine spirit'. This concept is defined by Jung as:

> The anima mundi, the demiurge or divine spirit that incubated the chaotic waters of the beginning, remained in matter in a potential state, and the initial chaotic condition persisted with it.[30]

---

28   Chodorow, 1991.

29   Jung [1875-1961], 1953-1979, Collected Works 8, para. 418.

30   Jung, Collected Works 11, para. 160.

To participate in the process of consciousness, Jung believed that we must dive into the chaos and begin to separate out the opposites. This separating process propels us into consciousness, for in differentiating we can see the nature of things: phenomena are appreciated through comparison. So in a Jungian framework a return to the '*prima materia*' is necessary for consciousness, and this '*prima materia*' may be found in the body:

> To neglect the body is to neglect half our world. It is to neglect from whence we come, the *prima materia*. It disregards our connection to earth, to matter, to the world of nature and to the feminine. Both aspects (psyche and matter) are needed for transformation. [31]

Clearly, Jung's view of spirit was alchemical, and announced a process of refinement of the '*massa confusa*', a changing of instinctual energy into a finer numinous property as Philosopher's Stone and individuated state.

Jung's concept of a process of refinement of the 'prima materia' has precedents in many ancient mystical traditions; for example, the transit of '*pneuma*' or '*prana*', a subtle form of cosmic energy, through the body centres, or 'chakras', in order to be purified. Whilst many of these theories of body and spirit rejoice in the body's vitality, I suggest that they often betray it in their emphasis upon its transformation into some higher quality.

I want to offer a non-hierarchical view of the transformation of energy in the body, valuing all manifestations of energy, physically-felt energy, barely perceptible neural activity, emotional energy and the imaginative processes of mind. I perceive them as different and complementary expressions of the same vital energy.

In our search for the meaning of our human lives we may long to suggest a purpose in the transmutation of energy from body to soul, creating, for example, the concept of a pathway to consciousness, bringing us closer to divinity. Indeed the plays of the book illustrate how embodied imagination is perceived to

---

[31]   Harris, 2001, p. 22.

develop self-awareness, interpersonal awareness and awareness of the divine or of nature. What we must resist I think is an overvaluing of human interpretation and rather nurture love for the communion with organic energy, which can help us to live our lives more freely and more fully. Psyche's journey with Eros brings her needs, vulnerabilities and dependencies into awareness. But part of this awareness is that she can no longer consider consciousness to be the superlative goal. She learns to give in to something more. This something more I link with the organic flow of energy present in nature. By awakening nature in the body I hope to find a better way to live. I believe like Peter Levine[32] that one definition of evil might be the restriction of growth. Stillness, movement, change and growth are the pattern of energy in the natural world. We need to take our place in this pattern to feel less hampered, less interrupted, less fragmented. When we block or control energy, we lose our way; we cut ourselves off from a source in ourselves and beyond that the ultimate source which is nature herself. From this rationale the body is certainly not inferior to the soul or spirit, it is neither cloak nor prison, it is the home of spirit to which we must return to find out how to live.

The relationship between energy, environment, body, brain and mind is discussed in recent writings from neuroscience. Siegel defines mind as a flow of energy and information[33] which arises from the interrelationship between the body, brain and environment. Cozolino[34] describes the creation of neural pathways in the brain, arising from inter-relational body experience which, once laid down, can either lock up or unlock creativity (an aspect of mind). He suggests that if neural pathways are created to allow us to function safely and unconsciously, then 'we feel calm and safe enough to turn our attention inward for contemplation, imagination and self-awareness'.[35] Thus the concept of body as physical ground for energy of mind is offered.

---

32   Peter Levine, 1997.

33   Siegel, 1999.

34   Cozolino, 2002.

35   Cozolino, 2002, p. 129.

The re-grounding of mind in body is the aim of much somatic practice. Whilst the definition of mind is various, the essential idea which pervades somatic practice is that body awareness brings self- and transpersonal awareness. For example, in Craniosacral therapy the intention is to dwell in stillness with the rhythms of the craniosacral fluid, bringing ourselves back to our connection with an eternal life pulse.[36] Or, for example, the Hakomi Method invites us to relax our will and to let a different awareness rest upon the waves of body movement in order to discover 'the happenings of the moment'.[37]

Transpersonal somatic practices such as these suggest that moment by moment perception of movements in the body helps us to perceive and receive energy from beyond the body's limits. We may experience sinking down into the body and at the same time awareness beyond the body. We may perceive our bodies to be connected to an infinite process. As one student writes:

> I experienced a connection with the earth and cosmos within my body. As I was allowed to roll and move infinitesimally slowly over the floor, keeping my eyes closed, so did I experience constellar 'echoes'. It was through this very gentle connectedness with the earth, revolving in a timeless, ageless orbit, that left me feeling filled with peace and wonder at the vastness of the cosmos within.

An essential starting point for the body's experience of spirit is the silent sensing of breath and blood in the stillness of the present moment. Mirabai, poet-saint of India, writes:

> In my travels I spent time with a great yogi.
> Once he said to me,
>
> 'Become so still you hear the blood flowing through your veins.'
>
> One night as I sat in quiet,
> I seemed on the verge of entering a world inside so vast

---

36   Boxall, 2005.

37   Kurtz, 1990, p. 3.

I know it is the source of
all of
us.[38]

Through such silent experiencing of body we may feel and acknowledge the energy inside, and we can allow it to manifest in movement. We have to soothe our craving to know where this energy comes from and what it means, by telling ourselves that experience without understanding can be food in plenty. Our minds must be quiet; it is often the habitual way we organise and interpret the world that prevents us from experiencing it.

In 1928 transpersonal dancer and choreographer Isadora Duncan[39] describes dance as 'the art that gives expression to the human soul'.[40] In 1917 she writes:

In my dance the artifices of dancing are thrown aside,
the great Rhythms of Life are enabled to play through the
physical instrument, the profundities of consciousness
are given a channel to the light of our social day.[41]

Duncan equates the 'great Rhythms of Life' with 'profundities of consciousness'. So too in transpersonal dance movement practice we find that by immersing ourselves in the rhythms of life we are left with a sense of being part of a profound process. As a dancer, Duncan perceives these 'great rhythms of life' as an essential creative blueprint for her art form. She experiences dance creation as organically self-forming. For Duncan, the purpose of dance is therefore to hold life rhythms in the body, as vessel of spirit, and the dancer herself becomes an expression of transpersonal creative energy.

1.2 Imagination is in the body

Energy may manifest in imagination, contemplation, meditation and empathy. These capacities of mind are considered in the

---

38   Mirabai, [c.1498-1550], 2002, p. 249. From the Penguin anthology *Love Poems from God*. Copyright 2002 Daniel Ladinsky.

39   Isadora Duncan, [1878-1927].

40   Cheney, ed., 1977.

41   In Rosemont, ed., 1981, p. 51.

field of neuroscience to be amongst the most recently evolved brain functions.[42] They are different from mechanical brain operations, for they are creative and intuitive, defying sequence and logic. It is often these capacities which enhance awareness and expression of spirit.

Contemplation, meditation, empathy and imagination may all be considered as forms of mind-energy[43] and they are stimulated by the perceptions of the body. We contemplate sensate experience, and we meditate upon, empathise with and imagine sensate experience. Our impressions of life are received through the channels of the senses, and memory and imagination seem to be able to re-conjure and enhance sensual and emotional experience.

Moving beyond memory, imagination not only revisions and re-experiences, but works creatively with memory to produce something new. The new version of the memory frequently focuses and intensifies the energy within the original experience: it gives a vision of spirit. Dreams may also be considered as visions of spirit, animating and guiding.[44]

The body is not only a perceiver of energy and sensate source of imagination, it can itself become a 'moving imagination'[45] or a waking dream. The body may itself be a metaphor,[46] a visible, dynamic and expressive symbol of human experience, holding the depth and the complexity of inner life and embracing relationship with spirit. The body becomes both perception and creative expression of spirit. As imagination fuses with movement, the vision of spirit becomes a live experience of spirit, having form, weight and dynamic.

In the dance with spirit, the body embraces many forms, patterns and rhythms. We may find that our bodies are attuned

---

42 Cozolino, 2002; Jancke, 2005.

43 Siegel, 1999.

44 Bosnak, 1998.

45 Chodorow, 1991.

46 Bartal, Ne'eman, 1993; Meekums, 2002.

with images of harmony. We become a butterfly, hovering gracefully, alighting gently, experiencing harmonious rhythm in the symmetrical movement of arms/wings. Or there may be other, very different forms, patterns and rhythms: the dissonant, the jarring and the destructive. The imaginative body can be wrenched and twisted by conflicting energies, hurled in frenzy, collapsed in abandonment. Imagination can represent the fullness of human experience and when merged with the body presents this fullness with movement and passion, giving powerful expression to the human soul.

1.3: Emotion is in the body

Connection with spirit stimulates the emotions, the passionate responses which we have to our environments. These passionate responses occur with our physical responses and may become imaginative responses.[47] Chodorow[48] charts and illustrates with case studies how the seven core emotions (fear, grief, anger, disgust, startle, joy, interest) may change into imagination of the mysteries, of beauty, of meaning, of relationship, of wholeness and the transformative dialectic of play and curiosity.

Joy and interest often emerge alongside the opening of the body through easeful, unrestricted breathing, relaxation of muscles, flexion and extension of the spine. Motion and emotion can encourage us into relationship with others and nature, and empathy and compassion arise from this relationship. Equally, fear, anger and contempt may be felt when the body contracts, tenses and withdraws, closing us down from relationship with others and nature, so that we cannot perceive and receive any presence beyond ourselves.

Our physical, emotional and imaginative responses are intricately inter-related. A layered response to our surroundings seems to happen in the blink of an eye. On the windy hilltop I may fling my arms wide open and lean my chest into the wind, I may

---

47   Chodorow, 1991.
48   Chodorow, 2006.

feel the emotion of joy, sensing and imagining spirit in me and around me. My body, my emotions and my imagination combine to bring me into relationship with life beyond my own body.[49]

Our capacity for energetic resonance, which lies in our bodies, can bring us into relationship with other people and with the planet. For energetic resonance can give rise to emotional and imaginative resonance, which in turn may create empathy with other human beings,[50] and with the earth. The body can bring us into contact and relationship.

The sensate experience of another's grief echoes in my own heart; I physically feel the other's grief and I am drawn towards or withdraw from (according to my mythic pattern) the one who suffers loss. Body and emotional responses may feed my ability to imagine how it feels to be the other.[51] Body and emotional experiencing brings me out of the shell of my own experience and into relationship. The barriers of self dissolve and I may become attuned to the other.[52]

Depth contact with another comes about when the body opens up to the presence of another. Claude Coldy's[53] 'Sensitive Dance' exercises educate body and mind to do just this. Claude tells us to let our bodies soften and open and to settle on another without printing or moulding. Hands become like snow falling on the other's body, settling on the other's form, receiving shape and essence beneath. This teaching of body gentleness, sensitivity and receptivity lies at the heart of the work described in this book. I believe it is these physical qualities that promote trust and empathy, and liberate our human capacity for expression and compassion.

---

49   Rogers, 2000.
50   Cox and Theilgaard, 1987, p. 174.
51   Cooper, 2001; Cox and Theilgaard, 1987.
52   Natiello, 2001; Pearmain, 2001.
53   www.danzasensibile.net

1.4: Spirit in body, emotion and imagination

In Section 1.1, I presented the body as perceiver and expresser of spirit. In Section 1.2, I considered how the body both fires imagination and moves with imagination, and in Section 1.3, how motion and emotion interweave. Here I wish to consider further the value of embodying emotion and imagination as transpersonal quest, and to show how body, emotion and imagination may dance together to create a passionate, dreaming body,[54] in touch with spirit. I suggest a fluid system, in which spirit, sensation, emotion and imagination are in constant relationship, transforming one into the other. I conclude that body, emotion and imagination may work together creatively to experience and reveal spirit.

In 'Turning point', written between 1911 and 1920, the poet Rainer Maria Rilke perceives that images must be loved if their symbolic and spiritual qualities are to be appreciated and known.[55] In this poem, Rilke tells us to involve our bodies and our hearts (our emotions) so that we may appreciate our images. Rational (separate) consideration is not sufficient to appreciate these images, there must be sensate and emotional involvement in order to receive the messages of the imagination.

Love and imagination are seen here as a way of knowing; we need to feel something about the images to understand them. Transpersonal research methodologies commend involvement as vehicle of intuitive knowledge.[56] Similarly, in transpersonal dance movement practice we enjoy the fluid relationship between body, emotion and imagination as pathway to spirit.

Dance may be propelled by the senses, the emotions or the imagination. Sometimes we find a still point in the body and we experience being connected to energy both within and beyond the body; then the imagination begins to combine with the body, forming shapes to express this sensate experience. Sometimes

---

54   Mindell, 1995.
55   Rilke, [1875-1926], 1911-1920, p. 129.
56   Braud and Anderson, eds., 1998; Moustakas, 1981, 1990.

the emotions deliver the body their passions and the body takes energy and form from them. Sometimes it is as if an image compels the body to reproduce its form. In all of these sequences, motion, emotion and imagination are in mutual, responsive relationship.[57]

Harpur[58] reflects on imagination as a 'different way of seeing'. He charts a history of the imagination, tracing the imagination to an ancient source in the presence of 'daimons' in the world. Daimons are described as paradoxical beings able to transform (shape-change) and pass back and forth from spirit to material world. Daimons, then, were physical entities embodying spirit. They were imagined forms of spirit made flesh, bringing imagination and spirit into the physical heart of human life, shaking us from torpid sleep, arousing our wildness and with it our human longing, hope and love. It may be suggested that when we embody imagination we ourselves become like daimons. Like daimons we physicalise an energy behind the surfaces of life.

When imagination is embodied, inner is brought into outer reality, and reconciliation, rather than tension, between the two, may be felt. When inner reality is fused with outer and received by others, a person will feel integrated and genuine in the presence of others, rather than split and hidden behind a mask.[59] Embodying imagination is therefore often experienced as a holistic practice, uniting soul with world, spirit with matter.

Embodied imagination has been experienced in this book as a form of gracious healing. This healing is attributed to three key processes: first, the experience of creativity, second, the experience of awareness, and third, the experience of connection.

First, the experience of creativity: when we allow and embrace the energy in our bodies, emotions and imagination, we wake up and surge forwards into life, unfolding, tumbling, being and creating. Letting our bodies experience energetic rhythms and patterns,

---

57   Chodorow, 1991.
58   Harpur, 2002.
59   Gordon, 1975; Winnicott, 1971.

letting our emotions express themselves and giving form to our images, all gives us a sense of being alive, of being animated.

Second, the experience of awareness: embodied imagination provides clarity by revealing the myths we live by. It lets soul speak through metaphor and so reconnects us with our inner life. It is in moments of symbolic authenticity that soul is stirring. This brings strength and direction.

Finally, the experience of connection: through breathing and sensitive contact with the bodies of others and with the earth it is possible to relinquish our fearful investment in separateness and to connect deeply with other people and with nature. This connection brings nourishment; it lightens the heart.

Creativity, awareness and connection lie at the heart of humanistic and transpersonal practice of psychotherapy,[60] as they lie at the heart of the movement work described in this book. Consciousness of internal dynamics is a primary aim of psychodynamic psychotherapy. But in humanistic practice, congruence (being truly and deeply oneself with awareness) combines with creativity to bring about self-actualisation:[61] an organic process of fulfilment of human potential in physical, emotional, imaginative, mental and spiritual planes of experience.[62] In transpersonal practice, connection with processes beyond the individual are perceived to feed and animate the soul.[63]

The fusion of body, spirit, emotion and imagination which ensues in the plays of animation and compassion in Part 2 seems to give protagonists a sense of their human potential: they feel awake and empowered. Transpersonal energy is experienced as a mighty force which carries them to the heart of their lives and the lives of others. It is like a calling from beyond: a voice which is both in them and coming from somewhere else. A cry leaps from the body as the mover scrapes and scoops the ground with her hands, her head bowed down: 'I want to grow; I

---

60   Rogers, 2000.
61   Rogers, 1961.
62   Maslow, 1976.
63   Moore, 1992.

want to grow; I want to grow'. This is both a personal need, and a transpersonal call.[64] Body, emotion and imagination are being called by spirit. By attending to body, emotion and imagination and letting them weave together, we hear this call.

---

[64] Thorne, 2002.

Chapter 2

Practices of embodiment and imagination

2.1: My starting point

I am in the dance studio at Tamalpa Institute in Kentfield, California. I will be learning from Daria Halprin (expressive arts therapist, writer, educator, co-founder and director of Tamalpa) and Jamie McHugh (somatic movement therapist, educator, AIDS activist and performance artist), exploring movement-based expressive arts therapy influenced by Gestalt ideas and practice. I have chosen Tamalpa because of what I perceive it stands for: dance as life, the body as teacher, the present moment. The Gestalt influences which I experienced in practice were: emphasis upon present awareness and attention to synchronous levels of experience (physical, emotional, mental).

Tamalpa Institute is home to the 'life/art process' which seeks to make 'rituals and myths out of common experience'.[65] Anna Halprin (co-founder of Tamalpa) has been active in communities, facilitating the expression and transformation of experience through the making of dance for decades.

As we interweave in the space, one participant moves towards me and holds my hand. She says, 'No need to fear' and I know that this is strangely significant to me as the tears come. Without fear we can go beneath the surface of things and touch the essential in the other, seeing ourselves, and realising we are all mirrors of each other and connected to spirit.[66]

Now we are sitting and letting our awareness hover upon our breath. Gentle, permissive, still. I am aware of a small weight resting on my chest, like a stone which someone has placed

---

65   Halprin, 1995, p. 47.
66   Trungpa, 1996.

surreptitiously upon my sternum. I take some time to focus upon this stone and I become aware of a contained (stifled) struggle between my breath and the stone. My chest continues to rise and fall, but with difficulty. My chest makes no protest, just continues to rise and fall as if it wants to ignore the presence of the stone. It wants to carry on as normal, as if nothing is wrong. But as I focus more on the stone, I feel its weight more keenly. It is becoming bothersome now and I feel motivated to do something about it. My hand moves to my chest and balls over in a fist. But it does not knock the stone off; it becomes one with the stone and presses down harder on my chest forcing me down to the floor. It feels oppressive now and cruel. Then I seem to turn into the stone, which transforms into a goblin, coughing and spluttering, louder now, from my gut. My body is curled over as I dance about, a goblin, wringing my hands and pressing down, down, squeezing and squashing, squeezing and squashing. My body is hard, armoured like a beetle and I have a tail, small and spiked. My movements are jerky, erratic and hostile, intent on repelling or damaging. Then I jump out of the goblin's body and I lie there exhausted. My face feels strangely open and unmasked. What has happened?

This improvisation was the starting point for my self-portrait performance at Tamalpa Institute. Arising out of my body, the goblin seemed to offer me guidance. It was giving me a focus for my performance as for my life,[67] showing me something I could not see. The destructive energies I was embodying were part of me and I needed to acknowledge them.

It seems to me that when something is ignored it has free rein to do what it likes, but when something is recognised it can be contained and balanced. Recognition without judgement seems to dissolve destructive patterns, leaving more room for life-promoting patterns to emerge and develop. This experience showed me how embodiment and imagination can reveal unconscious experience. Through sensing, feeling and imagination, I was able to embrace an aspect of myself which lay

---

67   Halprin, 1995.

hidden. The goblin: the destroyer, the silencer, the strangler seemed to enjoy this new recognition, his ferocity dissipated a little because he had been noticed. I felt awake, 'unmasked', vital, in contact with myself and others and the world around me. And this goblin had some energy, which could now be used creatively!

The guiding embodied image of the goblin let me experience powerfully in my body the hostility towards and rejection of self and others which lurked beneath the surface of my life. I sensed and felt the stranglehold this had on me. As I have worked with my goblin, I realise that he was born out of fear, fear of love and fear of life. In struggling with him I came face to face with my fear and I let him sit down and cry his losses away.

Energy for creative life was found through this cathartic and transformative dance. In the embodied stories of others at Tamalpa, the snake appeared frequently as guide towards vitality. Described by D. H. Lawrence[68] as 'one of the lords of life', the snake is a symbol of sexuality, sensuality and vitality;[69] that which is essential to life. As people became the snake, they died and then gave birth to themselves again, shedding their skin to experience a freedom of movement, breathing freely, rolling, organically unfolding, letting their bodies be moved. Dancing as the snake, these people entered a new state of sensation and awareness, more keenly aware of their inner life.

2.2: Authentic Movement and Dharma Art

Authentic Movement practitioner Mary Whitehouse[70] notes the difference between 'being moved' and moving. She indicates a process of giving way to the body so that it can move organically rather than be directed by thought. Whitehouse uses the term 'inner impulse' to describe the spark of movement arising deep down in the body, untroubled by choreographic or social judgements. Authentic movement is untutored movement, which frequently surprises the mover.[71]

---

68   Lawrence, [1885-1930], 1982.
69   Cooper, 1998.
70   Whitehouse, 1958a, 1958b, 1972, 1978, 1979.
71   Chodorow, 1991; Pallaro, 1999.

The process of Authentic Movement takes place in the space between mover (eyes closed) and witness (eyes open). Trust must be established between partners. The witness promises to notice her sensations, emotions, images: to be congruent in her responses. She attempts to step aside from her judgements so that she can behold a human story and an essential/transpersonal process.[72] The mover also promises to focus inward, noticing any judgements, concerns and thoughts, but seeking to allow the breath to awaken body, bones, muscles, organs, skin, creating a fertile ground for the seed of movement and imagination to burst open and grow.[73]

In 1979 Whitehouse[74] defines 'authentic' as 'simple and inevitable' and 'belonging to the person'. She writes of hidden movement which is the opposite of authentic, abandoned by consciousness, frozen, lost, vague, diluted. The process of authenticity is one of animation and integration of these lost movements; Authentic Movement practice is an invitation to notice them and to bring them into their fullness, and into consciousness through expression. Then they become an authentic communication from and of soul. Frequently images burst into consciousness from moving authentically, and such imaginative movement processes will be shown to you and explored in subsequent chapters.

The creative partnership between participants in Authentic Movement depends upon the partners' ability to identify and detach from judgemental processes. Human beings have a tendency to categorise, and to include and exclude others from groups of belonging. Judgements such as these work against the appreciation of our common humanity. Such judgements are usually made from the observation of external appearance and action. We seek not to find out about internal motivation and complexity, but require a quick and simple filing system based on superficialities. Such judgements therefore drive us away from the depth experience of others, and separate us from spirit.

---

72   Adler, 1972, 1996,1999; Musicant, 1994, 2001; Pallaro,1999.
73   Chodorow, 1991.
74   Whitehouse in Pallaro, ed., 1999.

In Authentic Movement, as in other forms of meditative movement practice, such judgements are noticed and attachment to them is released, so that we can sink deeper into the process of letting the inner self emerge through the body, as both mover and witness. The freeing of the body from the constriction of such judgements is an essential component of the process in Authentic Movement. If we can do this then the body is able to move according to its own nature, and the dreams of the body can be experienced and expressed.

When we sink into sensation with awareness (proprioception) we begin to notice movement in the body, normally unperceived. Our breath, our heart beating, the continuous rise and fall of our ribcase, the pulsing of our blood, the tingling vibration in our muscles, our skin, our bones: all this movement, normally taken for granted and ignored, can feed our imagination, animating body and mind.

The partnership of non-judgemental giving and receiving in Authentic Movement can evolve in many ways and through different processes. For example, witnesses may embody what they have witnessed; or both partners may silently make a picture of what they have witnessed in themselves and in the other, then share their experience with the mover as protagonist speaking first. The aim is always to speak from the heart and to own perception. Frequently, movers and witnesses find that they have made a profound connection with each other, that the boundaries of the local self have dissolved and both partners have become connected to a transpersonal mythic truth.

Authentic Movement practice has its roots in archetypal psychology. Mary Starks Whitehouse was strongly influenced by her own depth engagement with archetype as an analysand, and sought to facilitate emergence of archetype through movement. The Authentic Movement discipline, which she developed, may be viewed as a physical expression of active imagination,[75] in which archetypal imagery surfaces from breath

---

75   Chodorow, 1991.

and movement. The Jungian concept of archetype may be interpreted as energy[76] coming from beyond human experience, or as energy integral to humanity, spontaneously, physically emerging out of human experience, sometimes transformed into image. Whatever the interpretation, the experience of moving imagination in Authentic Movement is frequently transpersonal, taking mover and witness beyond the boundaries of personal journey and into the domain of the mythic: speaking of humanity, with its feet on the ground and its imagination soaring.[77]

Adler[78] eloquently discusses the connection between Authentic Movement and various experiences and perceptions of spirit, tracing historical antecedents of spiritual movement practice. As suggested in Chapter 1, Adler argues that the body, like the earth, is ground in which the transpersonal manifests. She perceives that behind all forms, whether they are images, music, sculpted forms, movements, or organic forms in nature, there is a presence and/ or process.

The discipline of Authentic Movement counsels us to wait until the impulse and the image create themselves. We are told to focus on our breath and to let the body be open to the rhythms which rock it. We are told to have faith in an organic process, ebbing and flowing in us as in the earth and the cosmos. Whitehouse's 'Tao of the body'[79] indicates a perception of spirit as process or way of things: for example the process of growth. The Taoist principle of non-action in action and action in non-action[59] underlies the principle of waiting in Authentic Movement. As we wait in stillness, a movement begins to grow. In Authentic Movement this receptive state is one of vulnerability and integrity, in which habitual ways of seeing are shed and faith is put in the organism as primary channel of the Tao.[80]

In Dharma Art,[81] a Buddhist art discipline, similar qualities are

---

76   Woodman, 1993, p. 151.

77   Rilke, 1902.

78   Adler, 1996, 1999.

79   Whitehouse, 1958a.

80   Whitehouse, 1979.

81   Whitehouse, 1958a.

82   Trungpa, 1996.

invoked. Openness, humility, compassion and relationship, all nurtured through the meditative body in the present moment, are considered essential components of awareness and creativity. Through physical experiencing of the present moment as we enter into relationship with the earth, we become aware of the interpenetrating and interconnected process of co-arising: the Wheel of the Dharma. When we feel this connection to other living things, the way things happen and interrelate[82] can be reflected in our art.

In both Authentic Movement and Dharma Art, a reverence for a process underlying the material form is present. The underlying belief in both is that the body needs to be in contact with this process to feel passionately, magnificently alive. Trungpa[83] suggests that by confining ourselves to an ego identity, we diminish our art. For art to become bigger than our own life, we must learn to connect with organic process and let it be reflected in our work.

Dwelling in the body through deep inner listening[84] and empathising with organic process[85] lie at the heart of the movement work present in this book. They are experienced as key tools in the conception and release of images into movement.

2.3: Transpersonal approaches to dance and dance movement therapy

The body has been honoured as a source of wisdom in a rich and varied heritage of transpersonal dance and dance movement therapy. I do not intend here to chart the evolution of the two pathways, or to offer extensive discussion of the perceived differences between them. My intention is rather to emphasize the points of connection and to give illustrative examples. Transpersonal dance and dance movement therapy are united in their focus upon contact through the body with something beyond the individual form.

---

82   Macy, 1991.

83   Trungpa, 1996.

84   Whitehouse, 1958a, 1958b, 1978, 1979.

85   Rockwell, 1989; Trungpa, 1996.

Before exploring the connections, I give a professionally-accepted definition of dance movement therapy (DMT). It is a form of therapy based on five theoretical principles:[86]

1.   The mind and body are in constant complex reciprocal interaction.

2.   Movement reflects aspects of personality, including psychological developmental processes, psychopathology, expressions of subjectivity and interpersonal patterns of relating.

3.   The therapeutic relationship established between the patient and the dance movement therapist is central to the effectiveness of dance movement therapy.

4.   Movement evidences unconscious processes in a manner similar to dreams and other psychological phenomena.

5.   The creative process embodied in the use of free association in movement is inherently therapeutic.

In addition, Meekums[87] offers a further principle:

> DMT allows for the recapitulation of early object relations by virtue of the largely non-verbal mediation of the latter.

Transpersonal dance movement therapy acknowledges all these principles and works with movement metaphor as a message from soul or spirit. As in psychodynamic dance movement therapy, the transpersonal dance movement therapist makes a commitment to receive the client's inner world in an asymmetric professional relationship, but this world is perceived not only as dynamically propelled by transference but as an expression of archetype and spirit.

In the therapeutic mirroring relationship, it is as if the transpersonal dance movement therapist, like the sculptor Anthony Gormley, allows her body to be cast by the client's soul.

---

86   Stanton-Jones, 1992, p. 10.
87   Meekums 2002, p. 8.

While the material is still soft, she awakens inside and animates the form, so that the client may see the hidden dynamic forces at play in the psyche.

In contrast to the asymmetry of the therapeutic relationship, amongst class members of a transpersonal dance movement group, *egalitarian* relationship is the vehicle for extension of insight. When each partner in an Authentic Movement dyad embodies the soul dance of the other, both partners meet each other on an equal basis, and each takes turns to hold the process of the other. This mutual holding of soul story does not occur in therapy where the therapist is usually paid to hold the process of the soulseeker, trusted as knowledgeable in psychological theory and as able to contain the sometimes volatile processes of the soulseeker's journey. I choose the term soulseeker for the person in therapy, as someone who is searching to embody their inner experience; this person is not perceived as ill, but as trying to return to the blueprint of growth and development which is a birthright.

Yet if we compare the therapist/soulseeker relationship with the transpersonal dance teacher/student relationship, we may find many parallels. Both relationships are asymmetric, professional and in both cases the therapist/teacher facilitates the awareness of the soulseeker/student through empathic, intuitive embodiment. I have witnessed delicate depth relationships in the context of transpersonal dance, in which students have become aware of the invisible through interaction with the teacher, participating in processes which might well be defined by some as therapy. These have not felt unsafe through absence of a therapeutic contract. Security sprang from the personal integrity and compassionate humanity of the teacher.

We may say that the intention in both transpersonal dance and dance movement therapy is to encourage creativity with the aim of experiencing soul. Creativity is valued in both as an awakening of potential. Kinaesthetic empathy in therapist, teacher and witness is experienced as a source of healing for both participants in the dyadic relationship, whether this is between therapist and soulseeker, teacher and student or witness and mover. Sensate connection with mythic experience heals the giver and the receiver.

Transpersonal dance and dance movement therapy are not concerned simply with local events pertaining to the individual, but perceive an individual's dance as containing humanity's dance and the dance of other living forms. In both transpersonal dance and dance movement therapy, we find a strong belief that our bodies can teach us things that we were never aware of or have forgotten in ourselves, in others and in our environments.

We may never have been conscious of our life energy, but our bodies can feel it. We may never have been conscious of our suffering in childhood, but our bodies can remember. We may never have been conscious of the suffering of our parents, but our bodies received it in the womb and carry it. We may never have been conscious of the pollution of the planet but our bodies feel it and manifest the effects. We forget our propulsion for growth, as we forget our childhood trauma, our parents' trauma, and the trauma of the planet. But our bodies do not. So if we inhabit our bodies and let them speak to us, we can become aware of transpersonal energy, and in welcoming it, we heal not only ourselves, but our families, our communities and our planet.

In transpersonal approaches to dance and dance movement therapy, we learn that our bodies can move in fluid, organic ways, and this speaks to us of our connectedness to nature; sometimes we learn through symbolic movement about our need for comfort, for passion, and for beauty. Physical, emotional and imaginative potentialities may have been overridden by the requirement to conform to perceived social norms of movement and being, whether this is conformity in dance or in daily movement habits. In both instances we are taught to switch off from our emotional and spiritual core and to copy movement which does not express how we are inside. We learn to hide our feelings, we learn to keep our strange visions under wraps, we learn to steer clear of our vulnerability and our creativity.

In both transpersonal dance and dance movement therapy[88] the intention is to reconnect with spirit, as energy, entity or process, so that movement is experienced as flowing from a source beyond human form. Transpersonal movement occurs in the public space of the theatre[89] and in the private space of the therapy room. If a compassionate performance community is created (section 2.5) then the empathy of therapeutic relationship[90] is present in the theatre. In both transpersonal dance and dance movement therapy, healing occurs through empathic witnessing.

Psychodynamic dance movement therapy[91] emphasises the body as container of memory (wounds are written on and in the body). The body is read for 'armouring':[92] muscular tension and rigidity; and the body is seen to give clues to the ego's defences. If these defences are experienced as problematic, movement is encouraged to explore them, and issues from the past may be voiced as body tension is released.[93]

Transpersonal dance and dance movement therapy also embrace the ego's defences, and seek to heal past trauma. But the trauma is not experienced as belonging solely to the individual, it is also about communities and generations and the planet. Transpersonal dance and dance movement therapy try to make visible the defences and then dissolve them through organic process, which is experienced as a healing process of growth: the healthy blueprint of the human being.[94]

Body and imagination are experienced as transpersonal tools, bringing wisdom beyond the rational mind. Anna Halprin[95] avant garde dancer and conceptual artist, describes the wisdom of the body in these terms:

---

88   Duncan in Cheney, ed., 1977, and Rosemont, ed., 1981; Mindell, 1995; Schmais, 1985.
89   Halprin, 2003; Jones, 1996.
90   Pearmain, 2001.
91   Stanton-Jones,1992.
92   Reich, 1933.
93   Schmais, 1985.
94   Whitehouse, 1958a.
95   Halprin, 1995.

The process of connecting with our internal imagery
involved 'dancing' the images that welled up from
the unconscious as another way of connecting the
mind and the body. In learning this imagistic
language, it became clear I was receiving images
from an intelligence within the body, an intelligence
deeper and more unpredictable than anything
I could understand through rational thought.[96]

In transpersonal dance and dance movement therapy,
symbolisation[97] is perceived as mythic and archetypal; the symbol
contains something bigger than the individual's personal story.[98]

In all art forms, symbol may be experienced transpersonally as
moving us beyond our own experience into a shared experience.
It provides a form in which to encounter shared inner reality.
Letting the body experience symbol means that the person is no
longer outside the symbol, no longer an observer, but the subject.
In this way, embodiment promotes empathy and resonance with
the symbol. To become the symbol is different from witnessing it
as a separate entity. When we become the symbol in our bodies,
we can no longer separate ourselves from its truth. It is us and it
belongs to us as it belongs to others. It is our heritage and we may
be able to accept it as a part of our life. In entering into this
process of embodiment, we are physically and emotionally
present with the symbol, vulnerable and malleable. In this
embodied state we can let the symbol teach us.

In 1917 Isadora Duncan spoke of the need for soulful
connection in dance:

It is here (*placing her hand on her breast*) that the
center of inspiration lies, and (*placing her hand on
her brow*) it is here. All kinds and conditions of
people have imitated my work. But they seem to
think it consists in certain stereotyped gestures.

---

96   Halprin, 1995, p. 65, Anna Halprin, *Moving Toward Life: Five Decades of
Transformational Dance* (Wesleyan University Press, 1995) Copyright 1995
by Anna Halprin and reprinted by permission of Wesleyan University Press.

97   Langer, 1953; Schmais, 1985.

98   Schmais, 1985.

In reality, it has its virtue in certain soul-states,
which are, in a sense, incommunicable.[99]

Mary Wigman's work was credited for its authentic
expression of human emotion. Martin, movement critic, dance
historian and author of *The Modern Dance* (1933) wrote:

The basis of each composition lies in a vision of
something in human experience which touches
the sublime. Its externalisation comes not by
intellectual planning but by feeling through with
a sensitive body. The result is the appearance of
entirely authentic movements, which are as closely
allied to the emotional experience as an instinctive
recoil is to the experience of fear.[100]

Other early modern dancers, such as Martha Graham,
transformed visions from dreams and dream-like states into
choreography.

The connection between inner experience and outer form
continues to inspire diverse approaches to transpersonal dance
in both Western and Eastern hemispheres of the world. In
contemporary Western improvisation, kinaesthetic, emotional
and imaginative experience[101] is encouraged through organic
movement. By paying attention to internal sensation moment by
moment,[102] kinaesthetic awareness is enhanced, and a 'handing
over' to the organic process of the body takes place. Movement
may then call forth images which complement energetic
experience, enhancing felt-connection with the elements of
nature, with the plant and animal world and with the human
emotional landscape. [103]

In her book 'The Knowing Body', Steinman discusses the
choreographic process of the contemporary performer Simone
Forti, whose 'zoo mantras' she describes as an 'act of empathy

99   In Rosemount ed, 1981, p. 47.
100   Martin, 1972, cited in Levy, 1988, p. 4-5.
101   Tufnell & Crickmay, 1990.
102   Blom & Chaplin, 2000.
103   Blom & Chaplin, 2000, p.11.

with animals'.[104] She shows how Forti begins to use her body as a source of knowing about the experience of animals. Forti spends long periods of time in the presence of animals, letting her body be affected by their presence, letting herself be possessed by the animal, so that her movement becomes theirs. Forti exemplifies the use of body empathy[105] in transpersonal contemporary performance, where the dancer seeks to know about and communicate the experience of others, both animal and human, through her body.

Japanese Butoh encourages depth somatic experience as a starting point for performance, which seeks to reveal human nature beneath the social veneer:

> Butoh starts from the premise that movement can originate from the non-pre-given, so you are asking the mover to go inside and connect on a deep somatic level. That somatic level embraces the neurological, the muscular and nerve functions of the body connecting to the brain, and also emotion. So the movement that can manifest through Butoh is very primal, primary, unmediated, and has a kind of authenticity and power which often eludes forms which are imposed on the body from outside.
>
> The task of the Butoh performer seems to be to somehow give form to the image, or that emotion is given form in movement. What is moving about Butoh performances as opposed to, say, a classical contemporary dance piece is the degree of surrender and sacrifice, a kind of willingness to totally open the body. There is no hiding, and I think that for an audience and for a performer is a moving thing.[106]

---

104   Steinman, 1995.

105   Cooper, 2001.

106   Rotie, 2005, in Smith, 2005, p. 32.

In Butoh the dancer engages with the image deep inside her body; she lets herself feel it physically and emotionally so that it is brought to life inside her. Through this process she makes contact with her invisible emotional potential: emotions which are taboo and hidden in herself, as in mannered society. She becomes a vehicle for their expression and release.

These examples show methods of practice in both Western and Eastern transpersonal dance which have arisen from a similar premise: that through embodiment we can experience raw emotions and startling images which transport us beyond our limited experience, into nature, into the animal world and below the surface of social interaction. When body movement is genuine: arising from kinaesthetic, organic and empathic experiencing, we connect with other living forms on earth and we embrace the depth experience of all humanity.

In transpersonal dance and dance movement therapy we find many pathways to embodying imagination. Here I want to discuss two starting points which are frequently present. Both require a particular state of consciousness, different from the active consciousness with which we interact day-to-day. I am suggesting a receptive, contemplative, unattached consciousness, which seems akin to the state of 'mindfulness' described by Hakomi practitioner Kurtz.[107] In Hakomi, as in other transpersonal somatic practices, and in transpersonal dance and dance movement therapy, this 'mindful' state is nurtured by an open, relaxed physical state. Our awareness of others and of our environment is enhanced by such a state. We are open to the transpersonal qualities of imagination; we feel deeply that the image is symbolic of something much greater than our own life. We are able to receive and embody images from established myths or thrown up inside our minds, and we play with them, knowing they are significant not only for us but for humanity and the planet.[108]

---

107   Kurtz, 1990.
108   Bartal and Ne'eman, 1993.

The two approaches to embodiment of image may intertwine, but may also be differentiated as:

1.   moving with an externally-given image
2.   moving with an internally-received image

In Skinner Releasing Technique, images are given to the dancer when she is in a relaxed, dream-like state induced by the teacher's voice and the inward focus upon sensation. The image is then taken into the dancer's body and imagination, and it begins to propel the movement. It is as if the dancer becomes the image and the image speaks through her.

In movement-based expressive arts therapy, as experienced at Tamalpa Institute, the mover is guided, through meditative focussing, to experience sensation in the body and to give permission to the body to move according to its own nature. During this kinetic process emotions and images arise simultaneously. We begin to sense and explore the image in our body, which becomes a moving metaphor.

These two creative processes of embodiment are essentially very similar. Both are receptive to the image, and they engage the dancer on multi levels of being. In one the image is externally introduced and in the other it is internally created, but both processes engage our bodies and our consciousness in an expansive way.

The essential quality in both instances is the ability to feel and perceive the symbol from inside our bodies. The paradox is evident: in going inwards we expand outwards. Through the sensual and emotional ground of the body, we grow beyond the body. Physicality is a key to expansion.

2.4: Courage and creation

Sometimes our courage falters when we begin to awaken and communicate sensations, feelings and images which have lain hidden. Embodiment and performance of dormant or discarded potential can only happen when we suspend our fears.[109] Many of us would wish to share the emotions and visions, born in movement work, but they daunt us. We wonder if we will be considered mad or bad, frightening or even dangerous. We fear that we might be criticised, shunned or even worse, imprisoned. And we may be scared of the emotion itself; it feels too deep, too raw, too awful; it holds us in its grip and we cannot speak it; our tongues are frozen.

To dissolve the fear we need much more acceptance of who we are and of what has befallen us. We need to embrace our fear 'as a sign that the creative moment is important'.[110] We need much more trust in organic process to see us through.

Body and imagination can help us to climb out of a disconnected, introverted, controlled and scared existence. Body and imagination invite us to live with spirit and bring us face to face with the process of creation and destruction in ourselves and on our planet. Body and imagination help us to embrace and fulfil our creative potential.

If we can befriend body and imagination, we can grow beyond the fear of our potential, because they can reveal to us a creative way forwards with the powerful energies which are present inside us. Tuby,[111] a Jungian practitioner, refers to the birth of a 'healing symbol' from expression and awareness of symbolic polarities.

The players in this book found the courage to experience and explore their emotions and images through their bodies. They were able to go through a process of catharsis: embodying, experiencing, expressing and releasing energy.[112] Through this process they found a momentary stillness and sometimes a 'healing symbol'[113] offering synthesis and inspiration.

---

109   McNiff, 2004; Rogers, 2000.
110   McNiff, 2004; p. 216.
111   Tuby, 1996, p. 34.
112   Halprin, 2003.
113   Tuby, 1996, p. 34.

2.5: Compassionate performance

Before I give you the plays, it is important to spend some time explaining the context of the work to you. Most of the performances on these pages were offered as partial assessment for undergraduate and postgraduate courses in dance movement therapy and movement-based expressive arts therapy. They were given to an audience of fellow students. The courses had emphasised process as learning medium which encouraged students to immerse themselves in their phenomenology both off stage and on. Performers and audience formed a community of people who were intent upon sharing their experiences through metaphor, keen to tell their story and receive the stories of others.

The context was one in which the arts were perceived as healing arts[114] and performance as healing performance, as in Epidaurus, the centre of the cult of the Greek god Asclepius.[115] Healing means 'to make whole' and the performance context of this work was one in which both performers and audience experienced the value of art in making whole. (The performances were sometimes experienced as a 'putting together' of self.) With this intention in mind it became easier to share, knowing that the deepest personal stories are the human stories, described by Houston as 'Great Story', and that in making myself whole I can help to make others whole too.

In dance and movement we often express our physical, emotional and imaginative responses to the world. Sometimes such expression is particularised and contextualised then claimed as 'mine'. There is a feeling that the performance makes a statement about the life of one individual; it belongs to the ego. In compassionate performance there is a strong conviction (rooted in experience) that my body, emotions and imagination bring me into deep relationship with others and with the planet; and that through the particular I make contact with the vast.[116] Compassionate performance is not only about personal myth but about transpersonal myth.

---

114   Halprin, 2000; McNiff, 1992, 2004.
115   Houston, 1987; Steinman, 1995.
116   Hillman, 1992.

This was therefore performance which did not seek to please, tantalise or entertain (performer and audience separated, in opposition); it was, on the contrary, performance which sought to promote empathy, understanding, communion and community.[117] In such a context it becomes easier to remain connected to our experience, because the performer is not being scrutinised, judged and criticised. Performance in this instance is not about artifice and cleverness. It is about a shared truth.

Anna Halprin writes:

> I don't want spectators. Spectators imply a spectacle that takes place to entertain and amuse and perhaps stimulate them. I want witnesses who realise that we are dancing for a purpose – to accomplish something in ourselves and in the world. We are performing our best attempts to create authentic contemporary theatre rituals.

> The role of witness is to understand the dance and support the dancers who have undertaken the challenge of performing. Spectators often come with their own personal aesthetics. They sit back and watch and judge to see if what is done lives up to their preconceived notion of a particular, very culture-bound idea of a certain kind of 'art'.[118]

Performance in the context of this book has been influenced by Halprin's thinking and by the experience of performance facilitated by Daria Halprin and Jamie McHugh at Tamalpa Institute.[119] Here performance never lost sight of process and authentic communication and the performance community provided a safe container in which participants could explore and share their inner experience.

---

117   Trungpa, 1996

118   Halprin, 1995, p. 249, Anna Halprin, *Moving Toward Life: Five Decades of Transformational Dance* (Wesleyan University Press, 1995) Copyright 1995 by Anna Halprin and reprinted by permission of Wesleyan University Press.

119   Chapter 2, Section 2.1

In the context of this book, performance is viewed as a service rather than an entertainment. Pinkola Estes[120] tells us about the Butterfly Woman, whose body is a metaphor for the earth and the sky. She bemuses her audience because she does not seek to entertain, but to serve, to bring understanding of the process of life and death. This is an ancient model of performance; it seeks revelation of spirit rather than egoistic show. Kuhlewind[121] writes of fear of performance as a form of egoism, where focus is on me rather than on the message I bring. In this book the embodied performances move beyond the personal. As the performers become rapt by the work, they lose their fear and begin to serve. Embodied imagination becomes transpersonal, in the service of spirit.

This definition and possibility of performance was able to happen because of the creation of a safe, bonded community for body and movement work. In the Prologue, I described this as the 'holding circle' of the group and defined it as 'a visual image for a united compassionate presence, which launches the protagonist in their venture to bear or suffer their truth'. My emphasis on the evolution of such community derives from my own experience of working with particular professionals using particular processes. Two key influences have been the practice of:

1. Jamie McHugh (somatic movement therapist)
2. Claude Coldy
     ('Sensitive Dance' practitioner: www.danzasensibile.net)

I will tell you what I learned from these two practitioners, for this learning has been a guide to me in the creation of the 'holding circle'. It is a challenge to write about the work of others and I want to be clear that this is my perception of their work. It is important to me to acknowledge their influence and it will, I hope, give you more insight into the context from which the plays in this book were born.

I witnessed a group, which Jamie McHugh facilitated, for people who had life-threatening illnesses/conditions. It was in the context of this group that I felt I learned a huge amount about the

---

120   Pinkola Estes, 1992.
121   Kuhlewind, 1988.

body in relationship and about the creation of community. By moving with people in confident contact, Jamie encouraged them to listen to their bodies and to dance out their stories. Through holistic relationship he enabled faint or barely expressed movement to flourish; he gave people the confidence to dwell deeply with their stories and to recreate themselves inside them. Through his involvement and his belief in the value of the work, Jamie facilitated the group to form a strong circle of engagement and compassion around each mover in turn. With this support, the mover was able to explore sensation and emotion in the present moment. The circle (sometimes literal, sometimes metaphorical) both held and nurtured the mover's process.

The creation of such 'holding circles' has since become a key focus of my own work. Participants have referred to the process and performance groups present in this book as 'a womb'[122] or 'a nest', images which convey the containing and generative function of the group.

My belief in the transformative value of the 'holding circle' has been further strengthened by attending to the practice of Claude Coldy.[123] Claude's dance practice 'Sensitive Dance' emphasises gentle, slow movement and contact, which respects the sensations, emotions and images of the individual. In slowing down and dwelling with sensation, we deepen our own embodiment and become able to perceive and receive the form and the energy of another person. Above, in 1.3, I have described the sensitive quality of touch, which Claude demonstrates and facilitates. It is touch which arises from a body which is open and soft, therefore able to settle upon the body of another without the need to form and mould; a body which can listen to the body of another and respond to it. If the body is hard and tense it cannot respond, it can only be adjacent. Hardened and clenched bodies cannot nourish another nor can they be nourished. A thaw must happen in the body for receptivity to self and others to occur.

---

122   Houston, 1993
123   www.danzasensibile.net

This learning from Claude has had a strong effect upon the transpersonal dance movement practice described in this book. It is through sensitive contact that intimate relationship is built. If such contact occurs in a group, the bonds between members strengthen, and the work moves to a deeper level. The preparation for the plays therefore took the form of much softening and thawing, through gentle exercises of opening and closing, curling and extending, receiving and moving with another sensitively and responsively. Like Claude, I ask the heart to speak through the body; for example, hearts are in hands and offered with care to the other people in the group. It has been my experience that the sensation of open-heartedness alters our psychic state; we share ourselves more fully and we are more able to perceive and hold the heart-story of another.

The movers and witnesses in the process and performance communities represented here were interconnected by being present together in a profound state of body and mind, in touch with invisible energy, flowing in them and around them and in the bodies of others. Such a state is described by Ruud as a 'liminal state'. It is a state filled with creative potential, in which movement and image manifest and disappear in continual organic process. The notion of such creative, connected community seems to have correspondence with Turner's concept of 'communitas', as 'intense comradeship'[124] and deep equality.

I suggest that compassionate performance arises out of the creation of such community. Compassion was defined in the Prologue as suffering with self and others, in the sense of staying present with experience. Transpersonal dance movement practice facilitates compassion, and develops 'liminal' community, which supports creative process and performance.

When we are witnessed by a responsive body (with or without touch) we receive confirmation of who we are. Cooper[125] suggests that we all have the capacity to attune to the body of another and to use our body's sensory intuition to perceive

---

124   Ruud, 1995.
125   Cooper, 2001.

another's physical, emotional, and imaginative experience. Part 3 of this book contains reflections by participants which support this idea. The body is appreciated as medium of depth contact with self and others.

Often during the practice of Authentic Movement, I ask witnesses to perform what they have experienced. Their bodies speak of the stories they have perceived, and their own stories become interwoven; both empathy and congruence are present.

Empathy develops by 'trying on' another's movement. As we enter into the movement, we are no longer separated from the other. Embodied reflection can feel more empathic than verbal reflection, less susceptible to judgemental processes of mind. When someone re-enacts our dance with respect, we feel strongly that we have been seen and not judged. This is affirming and nourishing.

The witness also gives something of herself in her re-enactment. Congruence is present in her dance, because she is honestly responding from inside herself to the movements she is making, given by her partner. So when she tries on the movement story she has witnessed, it becomes a reflection of the relationship between her and the original mover. The dance of the witness is about both partners. For in this new dance are elements of the original mover as there are elements of the witness as mover. The new dance can be experienced as a movement dialogue, and sometimes as a moment of unity.[126] These moments of unity may be described as moments when the witness sees and then embodies spirit, the mythic, the transpersonal.

The challenge of performing the dance of another is usually met with profound, sensitive involvement. It brings partners into a new relationship based on an honouring and appreciation of the other through genuine response.

When we meet with such contact and compassion, we can allow ourselves to be who we are.[127] Nurtured first in the dyadic

---

126   Adler, 2002.
127   Rogers, 1957.

witnessing relationship of Authentic Movement,[128] then in the expanded witnessing process of compassionate performance, the plays in this book are plays of the heart: they spring from the heart of the performer, and reach out to the heart of the audience. The process communities became performance communities as the audience witnessed and dwelt with an expression of soul in the theatre.

As the process of accepting the other deepened over several months, students learned to respect their bodies and the bodies of others as having something important to express about the wellbeing of the individual and the community. The final plays were experienced as 'Great Story',[129] binding performer and audience together. The 'holding circle' of the process community was strengthened even more in the experience of compassionate performance, as the audience witnessed and held the chosen creative expression of each performer. These plays were received as the quintessence of the performer's process, and such respect for the deepest part of the individual had a very profound impact upon the creative growth of each performer.

2.6: Live process into written form

I want also to tell of the challenge of *writing about* these plays of *embodiment*. The plays are no longer in the body and are transferred to the poetic domain; to images in words. They become a new form and are altered in the telling. Yet I persist in my aim, to recreate for you the passionate performances which I have witnessed. I believe that the written form may still communicate their passion and I imagine that the healing processes retold may still ripple outwards to you the reader.

So now, finally, it is time to give you the plays of animation and compassion. Will you come to these plays with a belief in the

---

128   Adler, 1972; Chodorow, 1991; Musicant, 1994, 2001; Pallaro, 1999; Whitehouse, 1958a, 1958b, 1972, 1979.
129   Houston, 1987

dreams of your body? Will you let your body be still, your breath softly rising and falling in accompaniment to the words which speak from the pages? Will you let reverie encircle your mind so that what you see speaks to you from another reality? Will you come into this theatre with me as your guide? Look, the curtains are opening, and the players are appearing before your own embodied imagination.

Part 2

Plays of animation

and compassion

Chapter 3

Mother and child

Hymn to Her

Let me inside you, into your room
They say that its lined with the things you don't show
Lay me beside you, down on the floor
I've been your lover from the womb to the tomb
I dress as your daughter when the moon becomes round
You'll be my mother when everything's gone

She will always carry on.
Something is lost, something is found.
They will keep on speaking her name.
Some things change, some stay the same.

Keep beckoning to me, from behind that closed door.
The maid and the mother and the crone that's grown old,
I hear you voice, coming out of that hole.
I listen to you and I want some more;
I listen to you and I want some more.

She will always carry on.
Something is lost, something is found.
They will keep on speaking her name.
Some things change, some stay the same.

3.1 Mother

This is a play about longing for a mother: a mother who was never known, but for whom a daughter's hungry body yearned. But the longing is not only for the physical mother, it is also for an eternal mother who will hold us and treasure us in her breast. 'Longing to belong' to the vastness of spirit is the subject of O'Donohue's[130] book 'Eternal Echoes'. In this play the longing for the physical mother is also for the 'divine'[131] mother; both are imagined as animating, reflecting, empathic, confluent beings. Moira writes:

> In the creation of my performance, I found myself going round in a circle. At the beginning, an image of my mother arrived in my imagination so clearly that I *knew* my story would be centred around her invisible presence in my life.[132]

Moira had experienced movement and touch in the 'holding circle'[133] of the process community with both bewilderment and joy. Students had been facilitated in awakening to sensation, in particular in appreciation of another's energy and form. Hands became receptors of another's essence, not seeking to mould and change, but to appreciate the other.

One exercise we do frequently is a sweeping of the body, making connection between head and feet, feet and earth. The hands of my partner settle upon my head and begin to contain, hold and encourage life in my body. Her hands gently sweep downwards, touching my shoulders, shoulder-blades, spine. My arms seem to lengthen as she sweeps downwards, spreading out my fingers, loosening muscles and joints. I feel my weight, I am heavy, massive; gravity pulls me down to earth. My legs feel strong and my feet rooted to the ground as her hands trace round the edges of my feet, helping them to appreciate contact with the ground.

---

130   O'Donohue, 1998.
131   Dadd, 2005, Appendix iv.
132   Dadd, 2005, p. 2.
133   Chapter 2, section 2.5

Moira was deeply affected by this exercise. It helped her to make contact both with the ground beneath her feet and the ground of her experience. Later she found herself falling and dropping to the ground; the ground became mother and home. In particular Moira was affected by the profundity of sensitive touch. This connected her to her most painful experience: the loss of her mother as a 10-month-old baby. For mothers often have the ability to attune themselves to their babies' physical and emotional needs[134] and Moira had been bereft of such contact. Perhaps the experience of this contact in transpersonal dance movement practice was all the more profound for Moira, who had lost this potential relationship so early in life. This contact became a catalyst for the unlocking of deep-rooted past grief. Here is Moira's poem:

To Mother

How could you do it, you must have been scared
as you turned on the gas and no flame flared.
Was it quiet, your passing, or did you make noise
as you slipped into sleep, spent of your ploys.
No more would I feel you, your skin against mine,
touching my soul in a race against time.
No more would the dreams of sweet summer days
enliven us both in deepening ways.
For I died too on that harsh spring morn
Yet free I was not to process and mourn.
Do you regret what you did, do you look down and stare
at the beautiful baby, abandoned and bare?

---

134   Stern, 1985.

How could you know when I needed you – you weren't
there.
How could you know what my life would become – you
didn't care.
How selfish you were, to deal with your pain,
abandoning mine again and again.
Oh what I would give for just one touch, holding me to
your breast – but I cannot feel you.
Oh what I would give for just one look, your eyes meeting
mine, soul to soul – but I cannot see you.
Oh what I would give for the sound of your voice
whispering my name – but I cannot hear you.
You are gone, as the embers of the fire cool into ashes,
as the sun from this day can never be retrieved.
And like the sun, you are eternal.
Like the moon, you light my inner darkness.
Divine Mother, you hold me in your arms, you gaze into
my eyes with love,
you whisper my name in the secrets of each breath.
We are one, all is well.[135]

This poem, born from movement experiences of sensitive,
animating contact, was the beginning of Moira's play. It speaks
of an utter deprivation of the senses, which long for contact with
a loving mother. As she puts the play together, she finds that her
body is wracked with grief. She writes:

From the depths of my being, tidal waves of emotion
began to surge through my consciousness and
'consumed' every waking moment. My body frequently
convulsed into sobbing, the salty tears of grief
outpouring their story of anguish. I was opening a
wound, stagnant and fetid.[136]

She dreads abandonment and exposure in performance,
which she locates in her original abandonment and exposure:

---

135   Dadd, 2005, Appendix iv.
136   Dadd, 2005, p. 2.

The fear of exposing myself in this way to the group shifted into terror, despite earlier healing experiences and my intellectual understanding of the benefits of the process. Dance movement therapist Gayle Liebowitz reiterates Winnicott's theory that an infant suffers unimaginably when she is deprived of adequate care from mother, giving 'rise to unthinkable anxiety'.[137] This accurately reflected my own circumstances.[138]

In performance though, Moira finds the 'holding circle' of the group[139] to be strong enough to contain the emotional content of her play:

I could absolutely feel the whole group's support and unconditional love. It felt easy to let it in to help me (very unusual for me!)[140]

During my performance I felt exposed, naked and vulnerable, yet, fascinatingly, equally powerful and empowered. The unconditional support and acceptance from my witnesses enabled me to stay fully engaged in the here and now, allowing my body to express her truth and at the end of my performance I felt wonderfully 'clean' and euphorically released. The group energy felt like a womb, facilitating my rebirth, enabling my emergence into new life. I felt 'held' by the group like a child held by its mother. It was a truly transpersonal experience, shifting me along my journey of transformation from helplessness to empowerment, from victim to master, from disconnection to connection.[141]

Moira feels that the compassionate witnessing of her play facilitates her rebirth. She experiences a physical image of the group as 'womb', 'holding' her like a child, as group members identify with the unfolding story through their bodies. This is a

---

137   Leibowitz, 1992, p.104.
138   Dadd, 2005, p. 2.
139   Chapter 2, Section 2.5
140   Dadd, 2005, Appendix v.
141   Dadd, 2005, p. 4.

reparative experience,[142] a holding in the womb of the mother/ group, a rebirth, and an embracing of Moira as the mother embraces her child.

In creating her play Moira finds that she is tempted to choreograph a variety of themes, taking her away from her original experiences of authentic movement. She catches herself doing this and commits herself to experiencing her loss in her body, which becomes a kind of dying and a kind of rebirth:

> The diversity of themes ultimately served to weaken and fragment the original core theme, which I later realised was an unconscious means of protecting myself from the feared reality of exposing my pain. So my myth came full circle to find me again, this time with a deeper, spiralling connection to the more focussed theme of death and rebirth – giving birth to myself.[143]

To Moira it was as if through experiencing the pain of her loss through her body, she was able to experience the shedding of grief and the transformation of this grief into triumph and joy. I am reminded of Joan Chodorow's[144] pathway to imagination of beauty and pattern. It begins with the experience of grief as a result of loss, conjuring the image of the void. Chodorow makes a link between loss/grief and absence of relationship to the body, sustained by lack of relationship to the parent. This seems to have been Moira's experience and now she begins to awaken her numb body, and with it the longing for the void to be filled by presence, presence of mother both earth-bound and 'divine'. Chodorow suggests that the body's response to grief is a feeling of heaviness, of emptiness and an aching heart, and that the body's reaction to such sensations is rocking, sobbing and lamenting. At the beginning of her play, Moira lets her body manifest her grief in this way. She allows herself to be in process with the motion of rocking, sobbing and lamenting until her grief is released and transformed into jubilation. She senses a pattern and a meaning in her story. She writes:

---

142   Clarkson, 1995
143   Dadd, 2005, p3
144   Chodorow, 2006.

Through my pain I am liberated. Through release I am free. Through opening my heart, I give and receive love, the agonising emptiness of abandonment now becomes fulfilled with the spiritual, creative space of clarity, insight and abundance.[145]

Moira uses masks to help her to connect with inner experience. She creates two masks: a mask of pain and a mask of transformation. She describes the effect of the masks upon her body:

It was as if they had an intelligence of their own. I was surprised at the authenticity which flowed through me as I surrendered to the overwhelming river of emotion that my pain mask released. Joyfully, my transformation mask released triumph and expansiveness.[146]

In choosing to allow her painful reality to live in her body, Moira is choosing authenticity rather than superficiality. This is why she feels 'fully herself' at the end of her performance. Moira lets her body live a till now invisible truth,[147] by breathing energy into it, awakening it and letting it express itself. This subjective sensate experience connects her to an existential longing for a creative, loving source, and brings her to the archetype of 'Divine Mother'.[148] Before her performance Moira says:

Because my experience was the only one I knew, I lived in painful denial for many years about the true impact my mother's death had had on me. All I knew was that I was searching to feel loved, searching to fill the agony of the empty and terrifying void inside me, searching to fulfil the desperate longings within, searching to know her, to hear her, to feel her, to touch her. Through many years of therapy and ongoing personal development I have faced many of my fears and much of my pain. I have been blessed with many insights and profound healing. This performance, however, is the first time I have ever

---

145   Dadd, 2005, p. 3.
146   Dadd, 2005, p. 3.
147   Whitehouse, 1979.
148   Romanyshyn, 2006.

expressed my myth with my body, with my whole being. My journey has brought me to this point in time, right now, to the edge of my fear, but also to the threshold of the temple, to knowledge, truth, life. Of all the cycles of death and rebirth I have experienced, this one (my performance) is the most powerful. As I address my mother and share my pain, I reconnect to Divine Mother. As I give birth to myself, I *become* fully myself. She (Divine Mother) fills me with abundance. I am rich in blessings.[149]

Here is Moira's journal entry at the end of the performance day:

When my time came, I was overcome with emotion from the beginning. It felt important to continue through the emotion and streaming tears (and nose!) and I felt triumphant achieving this.

Moving authentically happened effortlessly. It was as if the movement itself was leading me, not the other way round. I allowed the tears to flow and the sobs to release. It was as if my whole body was so relieved to be given permission to speak such profound truths, such raw pain. All my life I have been holding it all in, never knowing that I could give myself permission to release, indeed I didn't know what it was I needed to release. Today the time was right, it happened. It is memorable. Today I am whole. I am HERE. I have arrived. I have been born into myself.[150]

This image of being 'born *into* myself' (my italics) will be revisited in Chapter 5: Fire, when the play is of the Phoenix. The essential experience both here and there is one of embodiment, empowerment and creativity; through sensing, feeling and communicating my soul-self, I feel embodied and alive and I become creative.[151] Birth occurs in Moira's play through a kinaesthetic experience of self. The sensations and feelings

---

149   Dadd, 2005, Appendix i
150   Dadd, 2005, Appendix v
151   Winnicott, 1971.

arising in her body guide Moira towards this birth: a new and vital experience of self, an embodiment of soul. As she becomes aware of physical and emotional needs,[152] she expresses a commitment to seeking their fulfilment:

> It's like beginning again and I know that now I have to learn to suckle (metaphorically) and to communicate what I need.[153]

Having been born into her body, she experiences the need to 'suckle' and to feed. Nourishment is perceived to come from self-care (loving her body and communicating her needs to others) and from reconnection with a loving presence and a pattern in nature.

Jeanette Winterson describes art as 'an act of courage'.[154] I experienced Moira's performance as 'an act of courage'. It takes courage to reach down to the depths of the abyss of pain. It takes courage to sense and feel the losses. From the mud at the bottom of the pit of grief she emerges carrying her heart whole and held high. Since 2005 Moira has continued to research her myth of abandonment through two further performances. Her journey through trauma and the dark but fertile experience of anger towards wholeheartedness is charted in her unpublished MA dissertation.[155]

---

152   Gendlin, 1981.
153   Dadd, 2005, Appendix v.
154   Winterson, 1996, p. 99.
155   Dadd, 2007.

3.2: Voice

Caroline's story is one of finding her voice from behind a mask which has grown onto her face as defence against the pain of childhood. In a movement workshop, Caroline experiences the mask upon her face as she retreats from the drama. One of the players has become Cleopatra and Caroline flees from her impulse to lie at the feet of this imposing, maternal figure, so full of strength; and she, a baby or child so vulnerable and tiny in comparison. She needs the mask to cover 'the rawness and pain'.[156] Consciousness of the mask first comes in a preceding Authentic Movement experience:

> I wonder if I will move? It's difficult to keep my eyes shut against the light. There is movement, backwards and forwards, small circular movements; then my feet stagger forward; the movement is forward but reluctant, there is some hesitancy; my feet move first, then my torso and head follow. I have an image of an Egyptian hieroglyph, a 'frozen' statue in gold, then I see a mask, but I am inside the mask looking out. I can see the inside surface of the mask and am looking out through the eyes; there is golden light. I am wondering / thinking that only part (the lower part) of my body is doing something; I wonder about my upper body, then my arms move, upwards; I am not moving them, it is as if they are being pulled with string, like a puppet. I hold them at chest height, my palms facing inwards as though to receive something; as this happens, tears flow from my eyes. Something has happened/ shifted; I feel shock at what I am doing ... ' [157]

Development of sensitivity towards her body propels Caroline into an imaginative experience of startling force. The frozen gold statue and the mask are experienced as powerful metaphors for her experience of self in relation to her mother and in relation to others. The receiving of golden light, which seems to happen

---

156   Ohlson, 2004, Appendix 5.

157   Ohlson, 2004, Appendix 2.

despite her conscious self, brings tears. Later she writes a poem:

> In the beginning there was the voice
> And the voice sang
> But as the days grew and lengthened
> The voice learned it was not safe
> It learned to hide itself away
> It could not thrive in fire and ice
> In the frozen gales
> It hid away
> But left behind another in its place
> And the voice that spoke was strong
> To survive the elements
> A voice that drowned feelings
> An angry voice that shook the winds with rage
> With wild and screaming pain
> And time passed with the rage still burning
> Whilst far away the other voice was silent
> And the days grew longer
> Until ...
> Until the voice knew no other
> Until
> There was no other ...
> Then across the desert a wind blew
> Carrying a sound
> Silently
> Insistently
> Silently from far away but not so very far
>
> The raging voice
> Could not hear
> Amidst the noise and roaring
>
> But the wind blew stronger still
> Until ...
> Until the sound silent but loud
> Until ...
> The sound was heard

And the voice that spoke was strong
But soft
And caressed the wind with gentle words
And knew the value of time ... and sadness
Of tears and rage
Of memories and passions
It heard and felt the pain
Caressed the wounds and sounds
Of rage and tears
And cooled the burning hate
And said we are one

And at the end there was the voice
And the voice sang
This is who I am [158]

This song of reconciliation communicates the emotional landscape of the protagonist through the metaphor of the voice amidst nature. The angry voice which hides pain is reunited with the strong, soft voice of suffering; the voice which sings the whole story; the compassionate voice which sings of synthesis and evolution.

Playing with her mask, Caroline honours its value as protection, but is ready for its transformation into something less rigid:

When I tried to take it off, I was unable to; it was like trying to pull a very sticky plaster off a weeping wound. The emotional pain was intense and as I tried my tears started to fall. I could not do it; the skin underneath was too raw, the process of peeling was too painful. But a few weeks later I took the mask off and threw it onto the floor. But as soon as I had done this I realised that I had not given it the respect it deserved. I picked it up from the floor and rolled it in my palms until I had reabsorbed it back into my hands/ body. I am like a snake shedding an old skin. The new skin is relatively soft, but still affords

---

[158] Ohlson, 2004, Appendix 4.

protection. There is a sense of the old mask growing back out of me like layers of skin replacing and renewing themselves. The mask could harden again over time if I don't stay aware. But whatever happens it will never be exactly the same again.[159]

The action of ripping off, with the intention of banishing the mask, is not tolerated by the pain underneath. The pain and the mask need a compassionate response and the rolling and reabsorbing of the substance of the mask into the pain supplies the necessary acceptance: the pain is felt and the mask is appreciated as legitimate response to pain. The voice which sings of suffering the truth, is present in Caroline's body experience of the mask. She no longer seeks to destroy it, but accepts it as part of her being in the world. In so doing it softens a little, and allows emotions other than anger to be expressed.

---

[159]   Ohlson, 2004, p. 6.

Chapter 4

Earth

The clay of the body is energetically connected to the clay of the earth. It is this sensory connection which animates archetype. Spirit unites with matter to move the eternal stories of humanity.

In this chapter are plays of sinking down onto and into the earth beneath our feet, and into the earth of our own bodies. It is in the earth of the body that we find spirit, in the rhythms of the breath and the blood, in the momentum of physical unfolding. In Chapter 3, you witnessed a play of loss of a mother, the mother who briefly held us in her womb, and fleetingly embraced us in her arms, and you were present for the reunion with the eternal mother, discovered in the earth of the body. You also witnessed the child who had covered her pain with anger, and who found at last a strong, soft, inner voice, emerging out of experiences of authentic movement. In this chapter you will witness other new births of self, firstly as seed in the earth, then as rhythmic body. The sense of self as seed and rhythm is awakened through Authentic Movement practice, the still and silent sensing of self and the flicker of imagination creating embodied images in the darkness.

4.1: Seed

Wynona writes:

> In my family, the aim of life was to stay at the surface
> and survive. Deeply traumatised by war, abuse and
> poverty, my parents would find no good in the stirrings
> of the deeper realms of consciousness, and avoid
> the "underworld" of deep emotions, fantasies and
> mysteries at all costs.
>
> Such early indoctrinations form habits that are hard
> to overcome. Saved by a nervous breakdown, I
> finally broke through the crust of fear to rediscover
> my long forgotten spiritual and devotional nature and
> find glimpses of a flow of meaning underlying
> occurrences of my daily life.
>
> Giving attention to my inner experience, I discover
> that there is nothing meaningless, and that the Gods
> and Goddesses of old are still waiting for me in the
> dreamtime.[160]

Wynona reminds us of our own 'crust' of fear, a physical/
emotional phenomenon, created by physical and emotional
trauma. As our inner self[161] forms from sensation, emotion,
thought and imagination, it needs to emerge and be
acknowledged. Our inner self is sensitive to external hardship
and control, whether this is physical or mental. If we are lucky
enough to grow up in an environment which encourages the
emergence and expression of our truth, without ridicule, with
warmth and acceptance and joy,[162] then the fragile and delicate
inner self is able to emerge and spread its wings like a butterfly
in the sun. But if the reverse is true and we are met with control
and manipulation, the inner self prefers to stay in the cocoon,
which hardens ever more and becomes a prison, not a cradle.

---

160   Kaspar, 2005, p. 1.
161   Stern, 1985.
162   Rogers, 1957; Winnicott, 1971.

The inner self is intimately connected to the body.[163] When we feel emotionally and imaginatively constricted, our bodies contract and harden. Then we lose touch with our innate creativity; we cannot breathe nor sense the breath of spirit.

It is the reliving of a process of emergence which creates the possibility of a different story.[164] This is why the 'holding circle' for process and performance in body movement and dance is so pivotal to the outcome of emergence, as expressed in Chapter 2, Section 2.5. In a 'holding circle' there is no coercion inflicted upon the butterfly venturing out once more. It is a space of allowing and permitting, of acceptance and joyous witnessing.

Profound acceptance had been nurtured in Wynona's performance group through the discipline of Authentic Movement, as described in Chapter 2, Sections 2.2 and 2.5. The discipline had taught witnesses to be vigilant of the thoughts of the mind, grown from family and culture. Their careful filtering of judgements about Wynona's need for growth was important in allowing Wynona to emerge as herself; her previous experience of emergence had been sabotaged by critical judgement.

In the opening quotation (above), the imagery of underneath, below and inside is very strong. Already the core image of the earth is appearing. Surface life is aligned with 'survival': a desperate holding on to life, whilst the underworld is associated with deep 'meaning' and colour, through contact with spirit. The metaphor gathers momentum and seems to be pulling Wynona back to the earth, the earth of her own body, and her body as seed in the earth.

> I become a seed, encased in a skin, only my left hand putting out some feelers, I know I cannot move of my own accord, the seed has to be called to grow, awakened by the rain, kissed by the sun.[165]

In her imagination she has moved from the surface of the earth to being under the earth, surrounded by the earth. It is

---

163   Gendlin, 1981; Halprin, 1993; Rogers, 1961.

164   Clarkson, 1995.

165   Kaspar, 2005, p. 2.

from this new surrounding that she is able to feel her body and emerge again. The seed is a symbol of birth and growth. In the seed is a dynamic purpose which unfolds to express its essential self.[166]

Just as the seed wants to sprout, reach up and down, grow, change and die, so too the force of life, growth, change and death in us is strong. It was in becoming the seed that Wynona was able to sense the dynamic purpose of the energy inside her body.

The sensation of being a seed was strong and began to spark movement, thought and image. Wynona creates mind-maps to hold the experience:

called by life: sound
energy release: body
drawn by the sun: warmth, light
shoot
sEEd
root
collective records
ancestors
home: welcome, ground, earth
sacred place: love, be loved
sanctuary

growth: nurturance, affirmation, impulse
stem: strength
waiting: right time
potential
sEEd
containment
in-between: caught
underworld: resting
tied/ passive: bursting through[167]

The first stage in Wynona's life cycle as seed is the falling to earth, a movement which also occurs at the beginning of Ana's

---

166   Houston, 1996.
167   Kaspar, 2005, Appendix I.

performance (below) and of Catherine's performance (Chapter 5). This is a movement of letting go, and symbolic of decay and dissolution. It is a surrender to a force beyond conscious control, to a power greater than linear thinking can understand. Wynona writes:

> The seed must fall to the waiting ground, the old
> ways have to be shed, there is a death and surrender
> to the laws of change and transformation.[168]

She remembers and translates her favourite poem: 'Stufen' by Hermann Hesse, for her English-speaking audience:

Stages
(translation: Wynona Kaspar)

As ev'ry flower wilts, and ev'ry youth
gives way to age, so blossoms ev'ry stage of life
and ev'ry wisdom and ev'ry virtue
in its own time, and must not last forever.

With ev'ry call of life, the heart must be
prepared to say goodbye and start anew
and give itself with courage, and without despair
into those new, and different attachments.
And ev'ry new beginning bears a magic
Which will protect us, and will help us living.

Cheerfully we must traverse space after space,
not get attached to any one as home,
world spirit does not want to tie us down and curb us
it wants to lift us, and expand us, step by step!

Hardly we're settling into one of life's new circles
and growing used to it, inertia threatens!
Only a willingness to go on yet another journey
may draw us out of paralysing habit.

So maybe even our latest hour
will send us youthful on into another space.
Life's call for us will never cease.
Alas, my heart, say farewell, and be healed![169]

---

168   Kaspar, 2005, Appendix II.
169   Kaspar, 2005, Appendix II.

Now, as seed, Wynona is able to appreciate the earth holding and containing her in its dark womb. She lets herself enjoy the waiting, the resting time, before she bursts open and begins her journey into verticality, up to the sky and down deeper into the earth. She does not force the moment of birth, she waits till the movement comes of its own volition. The bursting open of the seed is a moment of authentic movement (similarly experienced by Joan Chodorow, 1991) when we feel that the body's movement originates from a source beyond our conscious control. Such moments are perceived as depth experiences; we seem to tap into a potential which is timeless and invisible but energetically present.

So Wynona waits for the impulse. She writes:

> New growth has its own timing; it cannot be forced or suppressed. It is a movement that has its own right to happen.[170]

> I found that in the stillness and the waiting, one of my hands wanted to move, slightly wriggling upwards, like feelers.[171]

She begins to rise and feels she is with Venus, the feminine principle, as she lets the movement reach its fullest potential, until the tide begins to turn and there comes the dropping down once more, the decay and death. The cycle begins again, and a new journey beckons.

In letting impulse speak in the body we find our way through the different stages of growth and discover themes embedded in each movement. Anna Halprin[172] has spoken of discovering a movement and letting the movement speak and develop to its fruition; then change happens organically, unforced, propelled from inside. This process was revealed in Wynona's play, as her body uncurls and reaches its full height, opening up to the sky. This opening then moves outwards and towards others as she invites her witnesses to participate in her performance. She writes:

---

170   Kaspar, 2005, Appendix II.
171   Kaspar, 2005, p. 2.
172   Halprin, 1995, 2000.

There was a high sense of energy and connection between the dancers.[173]

In opening her own body to sensation and contact, she encourages her witnesses to do the same. The play becomes a dance of relationship and compassion.

Wynona's play is an ode to life through embodiment of spirit. She lets her body be in the service of spirit. Spirit unfolds her and makes form of its own volition. In letting go control of her body, letting it sink down, relax and be held by the earth, she lets spirit awaken and speak from inside her body.

4.2: Psyche

The lost and found bodyspirit is the theme of this next play. Ana's process is to give in to her body and allow it to teach her; to re-find her self in her body, to let it move according to its own nature. It is a process of collapse, in which she lets go of her mental struggle to make things work, and allows her body and mind to sink into inertia. Out of this resting place, movement emerges and grows stronger, rhythmic movement bringing momentum and courage. It is the body which teaches this rhythm and brings to the mind the courage to carry on. In this process there is a humble submission to a force and power greater than that of the human mind. Through the body spirit manifests and shows its eternal rhythm.

Ana Rezende-Miggin writes:

> It was essential for me that during the sessions preceding the performance our group was led through a process that for me was about befriending the *stranged* body, particularly the feet.[174]

Ana describes how her appreciation of her feet grows during the preparation for the performance. She is able to let go her critical judgement of her feet and rejoice in their ability to help

---

173   Kaspar, 2005, p. 6.
174   Rezende-Miggin, 2005, p. 1.

her feel connected to both the earth and the sky. She writes two poems in celebration:

> My feet are broad like the roots of a large, tall tree.
> They carry the whole of me.
> In sorrow they carry my hopelessness
> Soul surrendered to gravity
> In joy they, my Feet, give me wings.
> The Gods laugh with pleasure when I dance
> Their breaths make me light as a feather
> The body surrendered to Levity
> Rooted and Winged
> My feet are generous.

> Feet
> Fire, Fast, Flow, Firm
> From the verb "to feet"
> I am feeted to the earth and I am feeted to practice!
> What a blessing it is to move.[175]

As Ana listens to her body, she feels a strong pull to give in to its heaviness. She writes:

> Being in touch with my sense of exhaustion posed me a dilemma, because this place of exhaustion in myself was about being paralysed, about not being able to move. The only way forward was to include this sense of paralysis. I decided to move the paralysis itself. As I hauled myself up from the sofa, I stood and allowed the sense of gravity to fill me up.[176]

Ana stays with the energy she feels in the moment. She lets her body speak. If she can let it be, then something will begin to change. This is an organic model, in which movement, like any organic process, must seed, root, fruit and decay and begin a new cycle. At this moment of process Ana stops fighting and allows her body to live its truth. The movement is heavy and takes her to the ground. She is surprised by the movements which emerge:

---

175   Rezende-Miggin, 2005, p. 1.
176   Rezende-Miggin, 2005, p. 1.

Including the 'inability' to move was a turning point in my creative process. From this point I noticed I handed the process over to the body, perhaps as Psyche gives over to the creatures that help her. I stopped thinking about what and how I wanted to present my myth, and trusted that my body knew my myth much better than my mind. I was surprised with the result, i.e. with the movements that came out and their meaningfulness.

I discovered a new sense of respect for the body, my body. I decided not to elaborate this performance in any other way. After 24 years I was going to give my body the importance and trust it was long due.[177]

By honouring the body, we let ourselves be open to spirit. The body can bring us close to the earth, and the dancing body can be in the service of spirit, making it manifest, bringing it into form. If we let our body move organically, its earthy heritage appears and it moves according to its nature, which is the movement of spirit.

Ana feels her body to be in the service of something bigger than her own story as she focuses on the message her body needs to bring to her. The movement sequence in performance is as follows:

1.   As Psyche, she feels overpowered by the enormity of the task. She can hardly move and falls to the floor.
2.   Collapsed, she gives up. 'Having given up, she can give over to another possibility, another potential'.[178] After a few moments in stillness, her hands notice her toes. Her hands begin to find out, 'Who is this?' She is discovering her body self.
3.   Her hands discover each other and their impulse to create music, to generate rhythm. Her body is momentarily enlivened by this, but she is not yet identified enough with this creativity. It frightens her and her arms collapse by the sides of her body.

---

[177]   Rezende-Miggin, 2005, p. 1.
[178]   Houston, 1987, p. 162.

4.   Something in her is moving. It compels her to get up. To live. It is difficult to move at first, but gradually it gets easier. Her hands discover her hips and clap against them. Once more a musical rhythm begins to emerge. This is strengthening. She walks more upright, her body beginning to loosen a little.

5.   She is no longer afraid of this force that emanates in the relationship between music and dance in her body. The music flows in her inner ear. She begins to dance. Her arms stretched out, her hands let go. She is letting go of all that has burned her up. She is letting things be, she is letting herself be.[179]

The movement process described here is one of letting go of the need to understand and control from an ego-state, a separated, individualistic state. Ana feels herself in communion with spirit when she releases her body from the captivity of her conscious control. It is through the freeing of her body that she finds a new wholeness of bodyspirit.

To find bodyspirit Ana needed an Authentic Movement process, in which stillness and patience were essential ingredients. She needed to empty her mind and let her body become attuned to its own song. Then her body began to sing and the music to reverberate around the ring of witnesses. Some wanted to get up and dance with her, pulled by the rhythm.

This play of new rhythm and life created itself out of the giving in to the body's need to collapse onto the earth. Out of this physical and metaphoric experience of earthy death and decay, new life was born, unexpectedly.

---

179   Rezende-Miggin, 2005, p. 2.

Chapter 5

Fire

Life and death are at home in the body. They dwell together there. The bird of fire, the Phoenix, brings this conjoining of life and death into focus in the single image of the nest/pyre. For this bird gives death to itself by bursting into flames and then gives life to itself by being born from an egg, which emerges out of its own blackened ashes. The Phoenix has become a symbol of the eternal cycle of destruction and creation, which we witness in the cosmos, on earth and in our own human story. Gaston Bachelard philosopher, advises:

> Should you wish to feel the marvellous tales of the Phoenix resonate within, you must discover the root image of the bird of fire in yourself, in memory, or in your fondest dreams. Lacking this you will travel widely in the fields of folklore and mythology as a mere scholar, learning more and yet believing less and less. The ever growing body of facts accumulated by the archeologists, historians of religion, and mythologists will lend your work an ever greater objectivity in accordance with the wise laws of archeological science. But this same objectivity, swelling with the number of well-ordered facts, risks to close you off from that side of yourself that dreams. This is why when a poem has been written under the sign of the Phoenix, one is inclined to see only mythological pastiche. A poem however must be true, humanly true.[180]

---

[180]   Bachelard, [1884-1962], 1990, p. 37.

Bachelard suggests that the image of the Phoenix was 'formed in one's earliest consciousness out of flaming desire to take flame'.[181] To catch alight, to be in the hot orange flame, to move and roar in the conflagration: this may symbolise our desire to live and die with passion and imagination, letting spirit fly and burn in body and mind. But to understand Phoenix we must become, as Bachelard says, 'the Phoenix of myself'.

Here then, is Catherine's discovery of the bird of fire in the dreams of her body. She begins:

> I'd like to tell you about the myth of the Phoenix. Once upon a time there was a beautiful bird and he was the most beautiful bird in the world. One day the Phoenix became tired and weary and his feathers began to drop off ... his beautiful coloured feathers, green and purple and red, all the colours of the rainbow ... only brown, old feathers were left and he knew that this was the time he had to die. So he flew to the top of the highest tree in the world and on that tree he laid himself to rest. And all night long he sang the sweetest song that had ever been heard. It was his last song. And when dawn began to break the Phoenix set himself alight.
>
> This is the story of the Phoenix [182]

As ever, it is a challenge to try to communicate the power of this performance, given with passion and generosity. Its strength lay in its simplicity and in its devotion to its own truth. Catherine wanted to embody the Phoenix, to imagine inside her body what it was like to burn up and die, and so to let go of the past, no longer clinging to memories; then to embody the rebirth of the Phoenix and to feel in her body its strength and splendour.

---

181   Bachelard, 1990, p. 39.
182   McLelland, 2005a, live performance.

Catherine began by telling us the story of the Phoenix as *her* story, for she was the Phoenix in this performance. Catherine is a visual artist and is drawn to sensual materials to enhance embodiment. She stands there enfolded in her coloured cloths, then begins to let them unwrap, leaving only black beneath. With charcoal she outlines the blackened Phoenix on a large sheet of white paper on the floor. Then she retreats to stand alone before it. Her voice echoes:

> I am the Phoenix. I have come to a time in my life when I have to die. I have to burn up in the fire. In the fire, I burn, I burn.
> I submit to the flames.
> I am the Phoenix; I fade.
> I fade into the blackness, into the ashes; into the darkness ... and I am gone ... [183]

She falls to the ground and whispers:

> We wrap ourselves in the black cloths of mourning, on into the sleep which has no memory. I die ... myself ... I die. We must mourn what is past, we must mourn. [184]

Then, her voice growing stronger:

> After the night must come the morning. I begin to awake. In the silence, in the blackness, new life begins to grow. Where memory scattered its seeds in the night, there is renewal – there is rebirth. In the hope of dawn, the Phoenix begins to transform; from darkness to light, from death ... to life. Out of the ashes comes renewal. Out of the ashes comes hope. To be reborn brings both pain and joy; in this, the Phoenix begins its journey into the light. Its wings sticky from sleep and newness, the Phoenix is slowly reaching; up to the light, stretching, reaching, awakening.
> Longing ... yearning ... aching ... [185]

---

183   McLelland, 2005a, live performance.
184   McLelland, 2005a, live performance.
185   McLelland, 2005a, live performance.

She is reaching now and she stretches towards her painting of the blackened Phoenix, and begins her rebirth into light. She touches the paints and her eyes flicker. Tactile and visual senses awaken. She begins to paint colours, slowly at first. She touches her face and begins to feel who she is. The pace of her painting increases, she is cutting open the tubes of paint, she is spreading and smudging, her body alive and in passionate creation. We, her witnesses, feel this animation as her body moves with the paint, body and materials swirling together as the picture grows and transforms before us. This painting process is spontaneous, flowing from the sensual experience of embodying Phoenix. Through her passionate body she recreates herself on paper.

Words are dashed through the painted wings and the fire. We read:

> You are alive, wake up
> Remember, but do not hold
> I am the Phoenix. I am alive. This is myself.[186]

Now she stands in the middle of the picture, and she speaks the words:

> This is myself. This is ... I, the Phoenix. I have died and been reborn, out of the ashes, out of the ashes. I, I am the Phoenix, I of new birth, I, the dawn of all new dawns. I am the Phoenix.[187]

Catherine is present in her new birth. Her face is shining as she clothes herself in brightly coloured robes. She looks into the eyes of her witnesses as she hands them ribbons of different colours. There is compassionate connection now with her audience, and we realise she has been telling us about ourselves: how important it is for us to reconnect with our bodies, to let our bodies sense the moment of decay and creation that happens with each breath, so that we escape from the numb pretence that we are permanent in form and move forward creatively into the potential of the present moment.

---

186   McLelland, 2005a, live performance.
187   McLelland, 2005a, live performance.

She is giving us ribbons, paint and brushes, inviting us to participate in this new birth. She speaks again:

> I clothe my new self, in colours of hope, in colours of life.
> Green for newness. Yellow for hope and for joy. For
> remembrance ... for all that is gone ... I will wear purple.
> For life and for passion, I adorn myself in red. I exchange
> my ashes for a crown.
> I am the Phoenix.[188]

As she imagines death through her body, she loosens body tensions, and with them the desire to control and hold on to the past. The metaphor of feathers dropping to the ground expresses the falling away of the old patterns. In fire we might experience such loss of tension as the flames lick the bones clean of the flesh. We, her witnesses, also feel light and full of life. We reach upwards with Catherine and we feel the colours pouring down on us and into us. We begin to breathe in the colours and we feel energised by her performance.

It is possible to view each moment of movement as a moment of birth and creation, and an opportunity for consciousness of spirit. As the breath enters into the body, the body is given life and can awaken into movement. To be present in this moment of movement is a challenge. For it is to be present in the eternally alternating dialogue between void and creation, unconsciousness and consciousness, formlessness and form. Keeping our present awareness with the air travelling down into our lungs, expanding them and affecting the rest of our body, we witness a moment of creation: manifestation of spirit in our body. This witnessing of organic movement can bring consciousness of spirit.

Performing the dreams of her body was not easy for Catherine. She was unused to involving her body in uncovering her emotional and her dreaming self. Of her process she writes:

---

[188]　McLelland, 2005a, live performance.

> The journey into my deeper self has been a cautious
> and reluctant one, but through the body I have begun
> to reconnect with my psyche: my deep and secret
> self ... The first of my dances was a cautious dance,
> a circular creeping tiptoe. My feet were like
> Russian dolls, one inside the other, my fragile,
> child-like self. In my second dance I was at the bottom of
> a long vertical tunnel, trying to reach up toward the light
> with my arms and my hands.[189]

Catherine took part in Authentic Movement processes with other students in preparation for this performance. Witnesses practised clearing their minds and making themselves open and receptive to the movement of the other. Aware of judgements and reactions, witnesses tried to set these aside and to perceive the core body communication of the other, the movement of energy in the body.[190] Then the witnesses were asked to go deep inside again, to reconnect with the perceived energy and to let it re-emerge in their own bodies for the mover to see. The witness's body becomes a dynamic mirror for the mover, catching the energy from the mover and letting it have life in the witness's body. Inevitably the energy creates an emotional and imaginative response inside the witness and this aspect of the dance is shared congruently with the mover. Sometimes emotions and images are similar and even identical; sometimes they differ. Such relationship was hugely significant for Catherine in being able to accept and share her own internal journey.

Through mask-making and movement Catherine begins to give physical expression to the dark, hidden aspects of her emotional inner life: the grief, the sorrow and the terrible rage. She writes:

> Through allowing these things to be seen, I have begun
> to acknowledge the self I have feared. This part of myself
> has been like a dark secret kept hidden: my 'mad woman
> in the attic'. In opening up, I have begun to see my image

---

189   McLelland, 2005b, pp. 2-3.
190   Chapter 2, section 2.2

reflected in others, and others have seen their own image in me. In sharing the unveiling of self, I have come to understand that others also have their secrets. I have come to understand the yearning in all of us to whisper, to shout, to wail and to weep over the shadows.[191]

Gordon[192] reflects upon the artist's need to communicate her truth, to have it acknowledged and received by others. This must be true for everyone. We all need to have our existence affirmed by the compassionate reflective presence of another.[193]

Through embodiment of imagination we bring our emotional life before another with weight and force. Our bodies and imaginations can communicate with great honesty, no matter how our rational mind tries to rein them in. They are always longing to breathe, move and fly according to their own truth.

In Catherine's performance, movement and image-making work together. In Chapter 1, Sections 1.2 and 1.4, imagination is explored as a visual pathway to consciousness of spirit, 'a different way of seeing'.[194] In this performance, Catherine makes an image from her body-felt experience. Her body becomes a medium of passionate identification with the death and rebirth of Phoenix, and this sensory/emotional experience feeds her imagination, propelling movement into an image on the paper.

The picture she creates is of a colourful bird surrounded by fire; she is:

A wing of fire, fire taking flight, a flying flame, the breath of wind that fans the flames.[195]

In being Phoenix, Catherine discovers an innate ability to feel, bear and express emotions both light and dark. As a result, she experiences herself as a passionate presence.[196] Her

---

191   McLelland, 2005b, p. 4.

192   Gordon, 1975.

193   Rogers, 1957; Natiello, 2001; Pearmain, 2001; Winnicott, 1971.

194   Harpur, 2002.

195   Bachelard, 1990, p. 41.

196   Natiello, 2001.

emotions are no longer locked up, judged as mad and banished from awareness. They are accepted and joyfully treasured as a source of vitality. In the imaginatively embodied conflagration, emotions take flight, burn themselves out and are extinguished. Out of their charcoal residue new feelings grow. It is in the expression and completion of a cycle of physical/emotional/ imaginal animation[197] that a new pregnant void is created. As each cycle finishes the sigh of peace and purpose is felt.

---

[197]   Sills et al, 1995.

Chapter 6

Stone

This play illustrates how material objects and the body can combine as media of contact with human emotion and with spirit. The play poses questions about the creation of performance and the possibility of authenticity in performance. But mostly the play is an illustration of the potential relationship between body and symbolic object in the creation of depth experience in performance.

> So where do we start exactly?
> I don't know! What do we want to perform?
> What can we perform? Can therapy be performance? [198]

Four young women have been set the assessment task of performing their process journey in dance movement therapy. They must trust themselves and they must trust their audience in this endeavour. [199]

They must trust that the journey into their inner life will not interfere with their ability to take part in social life. They must trust that vulnerability will be empowering, not dis-empowering. The process of trusting is always gradual [200] and requires a commitment to shared, compassionate witnessing.

---

[198]   Reed, 2005, p. 3.
[199]   Hayes, 2004.
[200]   Payne, 1996; Meekums, 1998; Hayes, 2004.

A mantra helped to create personal and interpersonal security as the group felt its way into the darkness of emotions and images: it was

> a chosen movement motif, to which we could return during the performance, if we felt uncomfortable with any emotions that the performance was giving rise to unexpectedly.[201]

To contain the work, a physical boundary of stones in a semi-circle was created. The stones were a symbol of safety. The dancers balanced on them and sometimes they moved them as safety was explored and experienced.

The dancers did not wish to expose their personal stories, they needed to keep them private. They preferred to bring with integrity certain feeling states which sprang from an 'inner impulse'[202] and to notice how in embracing these states they were brought into conflict or relationship with one another.

> By accepting how we felt, we were able to improvise with symbolic movements that reflected those states of being, and although much of the material created in those sessions wasn't used, certain motifs and qualities of movement began to appear as personalised movements to each member. For instance, Tracie often moved in a static, fragmented manner, while I tended to work with line and flow. Both Kelly and Amie often remained still, using gestures and head movements to 'speak' for their inner states. Through this process we became extremely familiar with how each other liked to move and could therefore start to complement that with our own movements; at times we even purposefully worked against each other's qualities and we found that this had an extremely powerful impact on the dynamics of the improvisations.[203]

---

201   Reed, 2005, p. 7.
202   Whitehouse, 1958b, 1979.
203   Reed, 2005, p. 3.

The group decided to explore the conflict between inner and outer experience; between soul and persona. Their process and performance may be seen as a journey with authenticity. They wanted their piece to reflect the difficulty of being authentic in public, and they wanted to show the tension between movement which sprang from the passionate and the heartfelt, and movement which was imposed and ingested. This was a difficult choreographic journey in which they often felt they had lost their way:

> Throughout the process of creating the work I doubted [the value of linking dance movement therapy with performance]. I felt angry and disappointed with my group because we were unable to create. I felt alone and frustrated in the presence of my best friends.

> It was only after we had given up and decided it was hopeless that the piece was born. Born from the despair and the hysteria, the piece took over our minds and bodies and created itself. Instinctively we all recognised at once that this was what we had been searching for ... I now feel a special, unbreakable bond between the members of my group.

> The process of creation was long and arduous; we choreographed multiple material and scrapped it all! Nothing felt true. The final piece was unrecognisable from the earlier choreographic attempts, but not separate from our process. Without the numerous failures we could never have reached this point. The piece reflected our journey far better than if it had been forcibly choreographed. It was the genuine result of a journey - the climax - a final release at nine-thirty one night that *came directly from within ourselves, and fed from one another* - an expression of our frustration, despair, disappointment, confusion and our underlying trust and friendship.[204]

---

[204]   Powlesland, 2005, p. 2.

In their journey with authenticity, they needed to find a form which would both protect and communicate inner passion and sensibility. In their efforts to do this, they lurched from setting material to finding phrases from Authentic Movement process:

> On the one hand, choreographed phrases felt false and insincere, whilst on the other, Authentic Movement felt too personal and 'inward'. It was somewhere between these two states that *Injected, Reflected, Projected Me* was created.[205]

The 'somewhere between these two states' suggests a place where inner experiencing and aesthetic vision unite, a place where inner sensations, feelings and images emerge into a symbolic outer form, changed, but energetically and emotionally connected to the original experience. The symbolisation of inner experience is oblique in visual/dynamic expression but deep in kinaesthetic and emotional engagement.[206] The symbol both protects and communicates; it shelters and reveals.

In the performance of 'The Stone', the two symbolic containers of inner processes were the metaphoric body and the metaphoric object, both serving as bridges between inner and outer worlds.[207]

6.1: The metaphoric object

The image which inspired the piece was a flower trying to get out from under a stone:

> My heart was not feeling strong and a large dark mass seemed to be weighing me down.[208]

---

205   Reed, 2005, pp. 7-8.

206   Cattanach, 1995; Winterson, 1996.

207   Chodorow, 1991.

208   Holmes, 2005, p. 3.

This image meant something to each dancer. They found a stone upon the beach and this became a resource for improvisations. The physicality of this stone was important because the dancers' hands could hold it, their feet could touch it. This physical contact engaged the dancers' bodies and from this physical involvement emotional and imaginative involvement sprang. The physical relationship with the stone was the starting point for an emotional and imaginative journey. It was a heavy, brown stone, which palm and fingers could enclose but not conceal. It was very 'ordinary-looking', potato-like, smooth on one side and scraped, slightly scooped-out on the other. The dancers began to play with the stone and gradually it gained significance in their work:

> The stone became a symbol of our burdens and oppression; burdens that need not be voiced but which could be expressed through movement.[209]

> The stone was not something we had intentionally used to become so significant but on reflection it was the centre of the entire piece.[210]

> We left the stone centre stage and as we began to edge backwards, all the emotions and energy experienced in the performance were left in the stone.[211]

> It was the stone that brought the group together and it was the stone that engaged the audience to feel a little of what we were experiencing.[212]

During creative process and performance the stone seemed to draw them together by receiving all their various emotions. Not only this, it seemed to act as a bridge between dancers and audience.

---

209   Powlesland, 2005, p. 5.
210   Reed, 2005, p.13.
211   Masterman, 2005, p. 5.
212   Holmes, 2005, p. 6.

The stone amplified an energy that was completely unique to the performance and became a channel by which the audience could relate to the emotions on stage.[213]

The stone seemed to contain contradiction:

Interestingly, while the stone began as a negative image—a symbol of our grief, as the work developed it somehow became a source of comfort and energy.[214]

It was amazing to learn from feedback that the stone was seen as a place of serenity and calm when in the rehearsal process it was used to contain the pain and anger felt by us as individuals.[215]

What had started as a symbol of a heavy burden, became somewhere to go to release, a vessel for exploration, a source of relief.[216]

The stone seems to have served two different functions. It was both a source of stillness and a facilitator for the expression of contradictory emotions. The dancers' bodies were stilled by the stone. They balanced and rocked alone and together with the stone. The stone was held in the palm of a hand, or cupped and caressed. When the stone was dropped with a crack to the floor, chaotic, jerking movements pulled their bodies this way and that. Somehow the stone and its loss entered into their bodies and as a result they became passionately present in their movements and emotions.

Perhaps the stone may be seen as a 'transitional object',[217] invested with the psychic realities of the dancers, and a psychic meeting place between the dancers and between dancers and audience. Perhaps the stone became a projection of their soul, allowing them to breathe soul back in: their emotions as well as their need for calm. And perhaps there is an eternal presence inside the stone, which touched them.

---

213   Reed, 2005, p. 12.
214   Powlesland, 205, p. 5.
215   Reed, 2005, p. 13.
216   Masterman, 2005, p. 5.
217   Winnicott, 1971.

The dancers were surprised by the heat of the stone:

> What struck us the most was the heat that emanated
> from the stone after the performance. It was as if all the
> energy, thoughts and healing occurred within that stone.[218]

After the performance the students placed the stone on my
desk, but I did not discover it until the next day and was
surprised to find it still hot. I held it in my hand and experienced
its warmth. Could it be through dancing their feelings and
passions with the stone, it became itself a vessel of embodied,
enshrined, 'enstoned' imagination?

> For me, the stone was the most powerful part of our
> performance/therapy. The thought of it fills me with
> mixed emotions; part of me feels tenderness and a wish
> to hold and treasure it forever, another part of me has the
> urge to cry. The stone became cherished due to the
> journey through which it guided us; it became a symbol
> of the past and a bridge into the future.[219]

The stone and the body were strongly linked in this
performance. It seemed as though it was through the relationship
between stone, body and mind that transformation took place.

6.2: The metaphoric body

The frustration which the group had felt in trying to bring
authentic movement into performance seemed to disappear as
the substance and symbolism of the stone entered both body and
mind. One dancer writes of being 'captivated' by the stone. It was
as if the stone charmed the group, held the dancers in a spell. The
stone seems to have precipitated the dancers into a physical and
symbolic world in which their sensations and emotions were
experienced and expressed in community with commitment.

Imagination was alive in the body, giving intensity and density
to the performance. Imagination fused with vitality seemed to

---

[218]   Masterman, 2005, p. 5.
[219]   Powlesland, 2005, p. 5.

bring the invisible into focus. That which they did not realise about themselves: their grief, their need for each other and for spiritual sustenance became tangible through their embodiment of and their physical relationship with the stone.

The dancers and audience were surprised, moved and changed by the piece. Here are some reflections:

> The performance left us all deeply connected to each other. We had found a deeper understanding of who we were internally and externally, and we had more of a sense of what helps us to cope with inner and outer conflict.[220]

> It meant so much to me that the performance was seen as 'fragile' and 'delicate' and that some felt something 'universal' in it. It was as if something beyond our conscious awareness was communicating through the movement, materials and music; something far more powerful that the words on this page can communicate.[221]

One dancer cited Lao Tzu to sum up her feelings on completion of the piece: 'Returning to the sources is stillness, which is the way of nature'. The dancers had let themselves be taken and shaken by the inner impulses of their bodies, bodies clenching and twisting, hands scurrying frantically over the floor, tearing up leaves. These sudden, jarring and sometimes violent movements contrasted with balancing, gentle rocking, simple walking, spiralling and flowing movements, and finally stillness.

A sound-score was created to reflect their improvisational and choreographic journey. It was a text of music and words which reflected the dancers' process of creation. It enabled the dancers to reconnect with their process experience, and served as a springboard for further improvisation on stage.

Here I give my edited version of the sound-score with dancers' rationale:

---

[220]   Masterman, 2005, p. 5.

[221]   Reed, 2005, p. 13.

1.   Voices off-stage talking to the people on stage, gradually becoming louder and more chaotic. Rationale: 'It was as if they were the conflicts and pressures which can send you mad'.

2.   Skunk Anansie, F.U.C.K.I.N.G. political. Rationale: punk music chosen for its explosive power and volume, its anarchy, and its confusion. In moving with this music the dancers were able to express anger, frustration and violence.

3.   Goldfrappe. Rationale: This slow, fluid, tranquil music created an atmosphere of contemplation and relaxation in which sustained inward movement could be found; dancers gave themselves permission to let their bodies move from inner experience, moving with or without objects placed on the floor. These objects had been selected for their emotional and symbolic significance, for example giant brittle leaves from the Eden Project and conkers were evocative of nature, home and family, scarves as symbols of vulnerability, entrapment and losing/finding the way.

4.   Voices of two dancers: 'Hello, is that you? Or is it me?' 'Are you looking at me?' 'Where are you?' 'I'm behind you.' Rationale: an inquisitive and contradictory dialogue intended to express confusion about location of 'I'.

5.   Mobile phone interference. Rationale: Chosen to show how external noise impacts upon us. Reactive movements were jerky and fragmented.

6.   Waves crashing, wind. Rationale: Rhythmic sounds from nature, chosen because they represented the balance and peace of organic life. The dancers moved freely and rhythmically.

7.   Heartbeat. Rationale: Chosen as a symbol of human life and as a symbol of return to the source of life, the earliest rhythm of life experienced.

8.   Ultrasound scan, echoing and then fading. Rationale: Chosen as a symbol of birth.[222]

---

222   Holmes, 2005; Masterman, 2005; Powlesland, 2005; Reed, 2005, gathered fragments.

The sound score reflects the struggle to find a home for the inner self in the outer world. Embodying and dancing inner and outer calling, the dancers experienced the tension between them; they became more aware of their inner needs and resources as they became more perceptive of invasive external influence.

Despite nerves, the group held on to its intention to stay in the moment with the material. The score, the set, the props and, most importantly, the stone were symbolic signposts for an embodied experience of the present moment.

Here are some fragments of conversation before and after the performance:

> I'm *really* nervous.
> Me too.
> I think we all are.
> We will be fine. We don't need to force it.
> Think of the stone.[223]
>
> Gosh I feel really emotional after doing that.
> Oh it was great! I really got lost in it.
> I can't believe it's over. All that for just one performance ... I feel like it shouldn't be the end.
> Hey you lot ... .feel the stone! It's hotter than ever before!
> We must have projected a lot of energy into it. You OK?
> I just feel really emotional.
> I know what you mean. We all gave a lot in that performance.
> Do you think they understand what it was about?
> Did we ever understand what it was about?
> Sometimes things don't have to be about anything, they just are. And that was! [224]

---

223   Reed, 2005, p. 12.

224   Reed, 2005, p. 14.

Chapter 7

Sea animal

The river is flowing, flowing and growing,
The river is flowing down to the sea
Mother Earth carry me, your child I will always be,
Mother Earth carry me, down to the sea.

The moon she is waning, waxing and waning,
The moon she is waiting for us to be free
Sister Moon watch over me, your child I will always be,
Sister Moon watch over me until we are free.

This chapter contains the embodied story of Merle. Merle is a fictional name, a French word which means blackbird. Merle and I liked this meaning because it links with the blackness of Merle's black horse, and it contains reference to body, for in Christian symbolism the blackbird represents 'the temptations of the flesh (its alluring song and black plumage)'.[225]

The sea can feel like our source and our ending. We may long for the sound of the deep sea-swell, its rhythm and power, or we may yearn to be in a calm flat sea, surrounded by miles and miles of liquid light. The movement, energy and light contained within the waters of the sea pull us towards it, our own waters rhythmic inside us, and dancing with the waves. In the water lies freedom. We gasp as the dolphins leap and as the seals swoop through the shining sea. Would that we could become as they, a part of the sea.

---

[225]   Cooper, 1998.

Merle finds herself transformed into a mermaid, far out at sea, sitting on a small island of rock. The group gathers round her and lays down shiny cloths and stones to create a beach lapped by the waves. We wonder how she is and what she is doing. Well, she is sitting and calmly waiting. There is a moment though, of startle. She knew she was alone, but then again did not know she was alone. And now that her aloneness is confirmed she is perhaps a little afraid. Alone, and a big sea surrounding her.

Merle, the mermaid, goes home and finds a deep pool of imagination in which to dwell. She writes this story:

> The waterfall was high and a torrent of water poured over its edge falling and suspended in the air. Sun shone through the falling water making each drop glow like a chandelier of sparkling light and colours that danced across the face of the fall – until the water hit the pool below.
>
> The pool was deep and dark and greedy. Consuming and sucking each individual falling drop of water, muddling them up, making them indistinguishable in the dark deep depth of the pool. There was no life; no current; no energy. Just deep, dark, cold, flat – a deep hopelessness. The water lay still and unmoving. Deeply cold.
>
> Further down the pool lily pads grew, and every so often, inbetween the green, flat, saucery leaves, a perfect waxy lily would sit on the water. Creamy-white petals and a yellow stamen; perfectly formed and somehow looking very self-contained, poised, elegant, dressed up and ready to go the ball – just waiting for the time to come.
>
> Then it came. Quietly from the depths. Not a ripple or trace to detect it. A face, staring. Unblinking pale eyes, looking through you – seeing beyond. Remembering, preoccupied, concerned. A ghostly body; graceful and

flowing, but moving fast, round and around the edges, searching and looking – ignoring everything except the search. Single-mindedly covering the perimeters, looking for a way out – a crack, a chink, a shallowing to get purchase; but nothing. The speed and energy lessens, slows down like an energy spent until there is none left. And motionless she sinks deeper and deeper into the dark depths. Deeper and deeper until there is only a shadow, deeper and deeper and then gone. Gone without trace.

Only those that saw her quest would know her existence. She exists for only those few that noticed her shadow in the depths and stopped to look further. Only those who watch and wait patiently knew [sic] the secret of the shadow in the pool.

Merle, 29th October, 2004,

Merle does not understand the significance of her story. It poured out of her, words singing up from inside her and written on the page. She finds an energetic but captured presence, a waif-like water nymph, searching for freedom. Merle does not know who she is, and yet she does know that she belongs to her, and is trying to tell her something important.

Immersed in an Authentic Movement process, Merle becomes a leopard. She feels the energy and strength of the animal, her arms and hands become legs and paws, easy, powerful and graceful as they pace. She is in constant motion, shoulders and shoulder-blades rotating as arms pound forwards. But suddenly her eyes are open. She cannot go on. She has been shaken by the heavy presence of the solid bars of a cage, which mock her animal energy.

It would seem that Merle's body and imagination are calling strongly for her attention. Given an opportunity to explore her creativity through body and image, she responds with joyful surprise:

> I found the freeing nature of movement literal and complete. The process and the pleasure of becoming physically uninhibited gathered momentum, overcoming conscious behavioural inhibitions. My journal records a feeling of 'letting go and indulging myself; I did exactly what I felt like doing and I really enjoyed it'. The concept of stretch and constrict developed this theme further and a feeling of power and restricted power was brought into my mind through my movement. When stretching 'my exuberance was wonderfully overwhelming, and I was able to skip and canter and stamp on the floor' (Journal). However when constricting my movement my steps reminded me of a horse held back by the rider. This feeling developed further into an image of a black horse, its head held down by reins and martingale, unable to toss its head; de-powered to make it more manageable. This image evoked memories of pretending to be a horse and jumping through the waves on the beach.[226]

Here sea and animal are present in the same metaphor; they belong together. As Merle lets imagination live in her body, the horse's pleasure in its freedom by the sea is felt in her body and in her heart. She then experiences the tightness of the martingale as loss of power.

Through embodying imagination, Merle becomes aware of a creative, passionate and powerful energy inside herself. It is pouring out from all her images, and these images take hold of her heart. She is in tears at the thought that the waif may not have eternal energy; that there may be a moment when the sinking in the pool becomes final. She cannot continue to be the leopard; the piercing eyes in its beautiful face see through and beyond the bars of its cage, but it is helpless to escape.

---

226   Merle, 2004.

Merle realises that in some ways she has not wanted to reconnect with her longing for freedom. She is bridled by the need to attend to her responsibilities, which have been separated from her creative life. There is a feeling of sadness here, but a need to carry on in the same way, because this is the familiar way. Longings are hard to legitimise when we are taught to ignore them from an early age.

Merle, the mermaid, is sitting on her island, letting herself be soothed by the waves, self-soothing, self-contained, trying to suppress her longing for the others to come and witness her. For there were others in the room, playing, creating, becoming characters, making stories. In turn we gathered round each person and found out more. Merle writes:

> There was something about 'not daring to hope' that the group would care for me and my beach in the same way that they had cared for others. I had definitely prepared myself for this by rationalising that it didn't matter, I was fine as I was.[227]

How often do we long for contact but tell the need to go away? How often do we yearn for soulful expression but banish the impulse? We push away from it because of fear or anxiety. Merle writes:

> When the group did explore my metaphor I suddenly felt scared, scrutinised, vulnerable; an introject of familial judgement.[228]

The fear is that the precious part of self will be damaged through exposure. This is a common fear in group process[229] but one which can be challenged and overcome through the 'holding circle'[230] of compassionate performance. So was Merle's experience:

> The group intention of warmth and lack of judgement soon overcame these feelings and I relaxed into the process. I

---

227   Merle, 2004.

228   Merle, 2004.

229   Hayes, 2004.

230   Chapter 2, Section 2.5

learnt that I liked my island; that I was on my own; that I was rocked by the waves; that I looked after and comforted myself; when I sat up I felt lonely, when I lay down I felt happy. I found that I was waiting for something or someone; I didn't know who or what it was, but I would know when it came.[231]

Merle the mermaid senses a 'missing element', the waif is searching for a way out of the pool, 'seeing beyond'; and the leopard glimpses life through the bars of the cage. In embodying these creatures, Merle experiences her deep need and longing for spirit, for freedom.

Whilst realising that something is calling her from beyond the life she has created, she feels compassion for her response to life as child and young adult:

Yet there is a knowingness that I am OK and I actually hang together OK... I have the hurt and the pain, but I also have the insight - which is far better than the defences I had put up to protect me. My life's patterns make so much sense now - and I smile at the very hurt, yet brave little girl (the warrior?) who took on the world, and became part of it, and created her own world (or island). It was an amazing feat.[232]

It is through the warmth of love and compassion that our icy, angry and fearful defences melt and our energy is released from captivity. This process has been witnessed in Chapter 3, Section 3.2, where the soft, firm, transparent voice absorbs the angry voice and the rigid, impenetrable mask is transformed into softened clay. Here too a thaw is happening, as Merle accepts her warrior's process of isolation, but knows that she is being called to challenge it.

Another vision comes as she sinks down into authentic movement. Merle is on a hill-top and her arms are swaying in the wind. She has tremendous strength and stature: an ancient tree,

---

231   Merle, 2004.
232   Merle, 2004.

with superb branches, moving sublimely, surveying her creations on the hillside. Then a different quality: a maternal impulse to soothe and protect. The movement comes swooping down as her hands caress and smooth down these small creations. She feels pride and love and fear. Then she turns her back on them, for she is drawn to go a different way. It is uphill, across a lake and then upstream and she needs a sturdy staff to help her in her struggle to find a foothold. The way is steep and it is hard to climb. But she carries on through the wet wooded undergrowth, up through the stones and the water. There she is called back from the movement experience and feels tired, exhausted.

Here, as elsewhere are polarised images: the wooded, stony uphill path is preferred to the open hillside; the waif desperately trying to find purchase on the earthy sides of the pool is contrasted with the waxy water lilies, beautiful, self-contained, waiting to go to the ball. On another occasion, making an image after a movement experience, Merle records:

> My drawing looks like warmth around me, arms hugging it in and a mist and warmth again on the outside. Yet there's a frantic look in the person. The figure is grounded, but has a desperate quality that I didn't feel during the movement. There are many arms. There is a warm glow around the person, and a warm glow on the outside, but separating the two is a cold coloured mist. It has trapped the person. She has a lot of arms, which symbolises my scooping and gathering motions. Why does she look so desperate? She looks overwhelmed, drowning; but I didn't feel overwhelmed during the exercise, I felt happy.[233]

This reflection shows how an image can wake us up. For the image is making Merle attend to an unconscious process. The trapping and the drowning are in this picture as in the pool, they are in the leopard's cage and on the island for a moment.

---

[233]   Merle, 2004.

Yet serenity and certainty dance with this panic and desperation. Whilst the serenity of the water lilies and the poise of the mermaid may be part of the defence of self-containment, they may still offer the necessary anchoring for the meeting with freedom. They may transform into determination as Merle begins her trek uphill; the climb is focussed but not self-contained: her feet meet the earth and she is awakened to the pulse of nature around her.

The creative state, which Merle and others have reached through dwelling in their bodies, fills them with excitement. It does this because it brings them into contact with a new potential, which lies dormant in much of waking life. Merle experiences a 'state of intense concentration and awareness in-the-moment'. She feels 'an openness, curiosity, willingness and trust to let go and enter a personal, and bigger, process.' Continuing, she reflects:

> It seemed *more* than a phenomenological approach, it felt almost like a 'walk of faith'. My feelings and actions were of swimming in the feeling and gathering it towards me. It was pleasurable, peaceful and there was a spiritual quality.[234]

Reflecting on Authentic Movement practice, Merle writes this poem:

> It feels like a mist, a fog.
> I feel it; yet it doesn't hold or bind me
> It surrounds me
> And cocoons me.
>
> Making me weightless, buoyant,
> Revelling and enthralled in the feeling.
> I reach into, and, dive in.
> I swim up – and dive down – and roll round and round.
> Breathing it in; more and more
> Like ozone; like smoke; a strong inhalation.
> An intoxication
> Of relaxation.

---

[234]   Merle, 2004.

> Of knowingness and wisdom that I cannot pinpoint
> Of harmony, congruence, synthesis, peace
> Of joy at the feeling of release.
> A kaleidoscope of past and present
> Merging, mingling.
>
> Of finding
> Of coming home and
> Acceptance in this moment.[235]

In Merle's process, the images are born on waves of movement, lapping inside the body and brought into form through dance. They bring her into a new relationship with the unknown, intriguing her with their physicality and their passion. They are like a waking dream, startling her and involving her emotionally. She notices which movements and images give birth to her tears, and she realises that this work is important for the life of her soul and her link to spirit. She writes:

> It felt as if something was slowly unfurling within me. I felt an openness that felt valuable, not vulnerable; I started to sense a new resource and potential within me.[236]

Trying to encapsulate what is happening to her through the work she wonders:

> It is something about: regaining balance between logic and creativity; a sense of potential, strength and personal power; feeling able to dispense with defences; and a sort of self-love or self-confidence starting to override historical antecedents.[237]

Merle continues to dwell with the dreams of her body for she feels that they are inviting her into the future. Reflecting on her story of the pool, she writes:

---

235   Merle, 2004.
236   Merle, 2004.
237   Merle, 2004.

When I become a waterdrop in the waterfall, my body feels positive, confident, carefree. I can hear and see friends, laughter, love and fun. When I enter the pool, I feel my shadow of hurt, sacrifice, disempowerment, judgement, isolation; my wounded child returned. The water lilies represent where I am now, and there is a feeling of personal alchemy, evolution, maturity, security. Yet there is still a 'felt sense'[238] of something missing – as in the mermaid metaphor.

The story invites me to the next step, to release the figure trapped in the pool. I suspect the pool represents my shadow, and the figure a trapped energy associated with emotions and material from my wounded child. Maybe addressing this will also remove the restraints from the black horse metaphor and prompt a conclusion to my 'felt sense' of waiting and of something missing – Gendlin's 'Whew'.[239]

We have come full circle, for you will remember the play with which we began: 'Mother', in which Moira dreams her early experience of abandonment, feels her loss in her body and her emotions and enjoys a keen sense of vitality in this outpouring of feeling for so long locked away. So too Merle senses that the waif's darting energy comes from an experience of wounding. Emotional pain, anger and fear contain a lot of energy, and through exploration and acceptance of these emotions, energy is released for other purposes.

In living the dreams of our bodies through compassionate performance we can connect with a huge resource of energy and creativity which may be sleeping, behind the forest of thorns, just waiting for our kiss. Merle experiences the 'polyvalence'[240] of her images, which carry her both backwards and forwards in time, teaching her about the processes of the past, and offering her new possibilities for the future.

---

238   Gendlin, 1981.

239   Gendlin, 1981; Merle, 2004.

240   Cox and Theilgaard, 1987, p. 42.

Merle's story concludes the seven plays of animation and compassion. We say goodbye to her and to Moira, Caroline, Wynona, Ana, Catherine, Kelly, Tracie, Amie and Sarah. I thank them for their honesty, for their willingness to perform the dreams of their bodies and to let them be recorded in written form. My own dream is that the plays have shown how soul can emerge out of bodyspirit, and how soul in one can reach out to soul in us all, touching our hearts and awakening our own yearning for evolution and expression.

All my life
I will clap hands in this water.
My body drinks in the mist
And my face feels the rain
Let me dissolve into one shining dewdrop
Let me be suspended
So rainbows shine through me
And my heart is as light
As a peewit chirping on a rock.[241]

County Donegal
August 1990

---

[241] Hayes, 1990.

Part 3

Epilogue: reflections and applications

In this Epilogue I bring the reflections of the participants. Their experience of transpersonal dance movement practice affected their lives and their work in dance, visual art and psychotherapy. Their reflections upon the links indicate the relevance of transpersonal dance movement practice for the arts and psychotherapy.

Chapter 8

Dance and visual art

In this chapter I discuss students' perceived connections between dance movement therapy (DMT)/transpersonal dance movement practice and creative process in dance and visual art. Definition of dance movement therapy has been given in Chapter 2, Section 2.3. Transpersonal dance movement practice can take place in the context of dance movement therapy and in the context of dance. As stated in the Prologue, it indicates embodied practice, which has absolute respect for experience of body, soul and spirit, and which has evolved from a variety of transpersonal dance and movement processes. Students' perceptions illustrate how dance movement therapy and transpersonal dance movement practice in community may be relevant to the creation of dance and visual art.

Most of the references in this chapter are to the undergraduate work with students of dance between the years 1996-1999, which was the practice base for doctoral research.[242] In these years, I did not ask students to make performances out of their process, because I wanted to find out if they made any independent connection between what they did in the experiential dance movement therapy group and their creative process. The analysis of the perceived effects of process therefore provides a useful, independent gauge for the relevance of this work for dance.

The data for this chapter are largely taken from interview transcripts (individual and group interviews) with 60 dance students from three separate cohorts, who experienced the work in the context of an experiential dance movement therapy group. This is a qualitative multiple case study, in which the voice of the researcher is overt, interpreting and organising the

---

242   Hayes, 2004.

data according to her perception and understanding. Subjectivity and relationship are enjoyed and also challenged as sources of understanding, and the researcher invites dialogue with other researchers of process and practice in the arts and therapy.

In each cohort, the experiential dance movement therapy group took place weekly over a period of ten weeks. Each session lasted ninety minutes and involved sixty minutes of warm-up and improvisational process with music and props (for example, large stretchy cloths of lycra) and thirty minutes of verbal processing. The differences between experiential dance movement therapy and dance movement therapy involving therapeutic relationship were clearly defined. Students understood that they would experience as learners the simple formula of a dance movement therapy group session (the circular warm-up highlighting connections between movement and emotion, followed by an open exploratory process) as taught on the Laban MA in Dance Movement Therapy (1990-1993). They knew that the facilitator would not enter into therapeutic relationship with individuals (working actively with arising issues), but would aim to encourage expression and responsibility in this community of learners.

This chapter uses the undergraduate study as a springboard for discussion of the relevance of experiential dance movement therapy and transpersonal dance movement practice for dance and visual art. In particular, the undergraduate students' responses to the question: 'Has your experience of dance movement therapy affected your creative work at university?' have been used to create a pathway for discussion.

Since the doctoral study, my work has become increasingly transpersonal, and I have redefined my practice accordingly. Visual artists and dancers on postgraduate programmes as well as subsequent undergraduate dance students who have participated in transpersonal dance movement practice are also represented in this chapter, with reference to interviews and questionnaires. These students were given the opportunity to perform the dreams of their bodies in plays of animation and compassion as part of their assessment. Some of their plays are in Part 2.

First I will look at students' perceived outcomes of the work, then I will examine the perceived application of these outcomes to creative work in dance and visual art. In synopsis, the perceived outcomes of experiential dance movement therapy in the undergraduate study were threefold. Student dancers felt an increase in playfulness, in self-confidence and in relationship. These three terms were chosen to hold and describe the outcomes of the work in the undergraduate study[243] and they provide a useful foundation for discussion of the work on postgraduate programmes, as well as subsequent undergraduate work.

The term 'playfulness' encompasses spontaneity, receptivity and creativity. It was chosen to communicate the sense of fluidity and openness in body and imagination which participants experienced and expressed. Self-confidence has many layers and refers here to a sense of cherished existence in self as separate body and soul[244] and in self as bodyspirit. Relationship refers to a sense of connection to our own body, emotions, images and thoughts, to the bodies of others and to their internal worlds, as well as to earth, nature and cosmos. It therefore describes an increased sense of relatedness and belonging on many levels. Whilst these three concepts are discussed independently below, they are perceived as intertwining. For playfulness and self-confidence mutually fertilise each other (when we become more playful, we feel more self-confident; when we become more self-confident, we are more able to play), as do self-confidence and relationship (when we trust and delight more in ourselves, this brings us into relationship, and through relationship we come to accept ourselves more readily), as do relationship and playfulness (relationship can be promoted through play, and playfulness may be developed through responsive relationship[245]). These connections will reveal themselves as I discuss the concepts in the context of creativity in the arts of dance and visual art.

---

243   Hayes, 2004.
244   Stern, 1985.
245   Winnicott, 1971.

8.1 Playfulness, dance and visual art

The undergraduate study

The dancers who took part in the undergraduate study believed that the playfulness of experiential dance movement therapy had enhanced their creative process in different ways, in terms of content, quality of movement, relaxation, revitalisation, receptivity and choreographic process. Here is an example of how content was used directly as a resource for choreography and performance:

> In the experiential group that week the music and movement were really slow and ambient, sort of sunny and I imagined feeling really happy and relaxed. Everyone's movements were soft and wave-like, and upward, like a utopia. I've transferred this moment to my choreography, when C has a shiny lilac cloth wrapped around her and she's moving slowly, wave-like, it's like she's being born, coming out of a cocoon.

Relational dynamics, being presented in performance, were explored in experiential dance movement therapy:

> In the session I was dragging X around. I felt I was being really manipulative. I was dragging her and taking her where I wanted to and she was doing what I wanted her to do and I had a sense of being in control because in my own life I'm really quite weak in the sense that I'll always do things for other people to please them… My dissertation is closely connected to me because I'm looking at Greek dance and gender roles. [Movement] for the men is bigger and more fancy, whereas the women are more restricted in their movement. Through my upbringing I've been very restricted.

This exploration seems to have deepened emotional understanding of the dynamics of control and resistance, power and restriction which affected choreographic intention and decision.

Generally, experiential dance movement therapy gave students an opportunity to explore their choreographic themes subjectively, deepening their understanding of cultural, social patterns of behaviour, and the effects on the inner life of the individual. This identification with the subject matter was perceived as giving their choreography and performance more integrity and credibility. Several themes alive in the experiential dance movement therapy group (such as restriction, safety, escape and belonging), and therefore explored subjectively, were considered to be relevant and helpful to the maturation of choreographic themes.

The movement quality in experiential dance movement therapy was described variously as 'playful', 'organic', 'flowing', 'spontaneous', 'connected to feeling', 'empowering', 'dynamic' 'alive'. Several participants spoke about the transfer of movement quality from experiential dance movement therapy to technique and choreography:

> I used to have a bit of a problem with balance, but it seems to flow now; I just feel free, I noticed a difference. It wasn't just dance, it was me as well. Whether it looked fluid or not I don't know, but I felt fluid and I felt I was not under pressure. I was able to enjoy it and wanting to carry on and not wanting the class to end.

Participants reflected on the benefit of relaxation of their analytic aesthetic consciousness in enhancing their creative ability. They felt that the joy of experiential dance movement therapy for them had been its separateness from choreographic agendas. It had been a context in which they could forget about aesthetics, relax and let go of 'left-brain thinking'. They felt that they could enjoy 'experiencing', rather than 'analysing': 'Having the time to move without any constraints, not necessarily thinking about things but just exploring'. This expansive, playful attitude was perceived as developing creative possibility: 'I'm not so serious in the experiential group. I can be funny; I can be many things'.

So experiential dance movement therapy was experienced as creatively replenishing. In many cases the experience of dance movement therapy brought back positive memories of childhood, its freedom and its spontaneity. Many participants spoke of feeling refreshed and inspired by this reconnection with childhood. Generally, through participation in experiential dance movement therapy, dancers felt more 'open' and 'free' to take risks and explore new ways of working with material, sometimes using media they had not worked with before.

Playfulness was described as 'an openness to spirit' by some dancers. They experienced moments of 'being moved'[246] by an energy beyond their conscious awareness: moments when their body received form and dynamic in surprising ways. They experienced being pulled to the ground or being lifted outwards and upwards. This experience of being moved was perceived as bringing dancers closer to spirit, investing their work with transpersonal significance.

Many participants transferred their experience of playfulness in experiential dance movement therapy to choreographic process:

> We spent eight weeks as a whole group, working up to the performance. Each group would be like a therapy session in a way. We would 'jam', improvising all session, you could do what you want, you didn't have to move and you could speak if you wanted to.

They found that playing helped to generate movement which was meaningful for the dancers, and that such movement, when recreated in performance, held the spark of its genesis.

Postgraduate and subsequent undergraduate work

Recently, a visual artist involved in the postgraduate study described to me how she transferred practice from Authentic Movement to image-making. She relaxed her body and quietened

---

246   Whitehouse, 1958a, 1958b, 1979.

her mind by closing her eyes and focussing on physical sensation. Then, standing before her paper, with charcoal in her hands, she waited for the movements to come, letting these movements make the marks on the paper, without seeing the forms and without judging them. Her arm movements arose from swaying and bending her upper body in response to her breathing in and out. She was delighted and intrigued with what was created: an image, containing un-thought of shapes and momentum, which had made itself through her animated body.

The relationship between receiving and designing form has been discussed extensively in dance literature[247] as elsewhere, and it is suggested here that creative process requires an ability to blend receptivity with aesthetic skill. Receptivity is a quality which arises from the ability to perceive through our senses. It involves an active awakening of our perceptual abilities. If we can become aware of sensation, emotion and image as they arise inside us, we can use these movements and forms as resources in our conscious definition of form.

It has been suggested that receptivity and playfulness are synonymous, for in playing we are open to creative possibilities emerging through sensation, emotion and image. Meekums[248] emphasizes the importance of play in creative process. She suggests the cultivation of a hovering attention to spontaneously forming movement and imagination as creative choices are made.

Playfulness here suggests a movement process in dance, which embraces and explores imagery and ideas as they emerge, as well as a choreographic process, which tries out ideas without fixity and attachment. In the postgraduate work there were many examples of students playing with movement and image-making, waiting to see what would emerge. Whilst there was no aesthetic intention behind this process, they found that it frequently threw up material which ignited and resourced their art.

---

247   For example, Beiswanger, 1962, Nadel and Nadel Miller, 1978.

248   Meekums, 1993.

When we play, we do not know what is going to happen. We surrender our will to the dynamics of the moment. We respond to these with our organic, spontaneous self, participating in a 'here and now' process. With reference to music improvisation, Paton[249] describes the change from conscious to receptive process, citing Ruud:[250]

> This suggests a model of the imagination, in which unconscious and conscious processes work together to create original outcomes. Whilst an improvisation might begin with a consciously applied structure, there is always a moment when the music moves into another, less conscious mode of performance...This suggests an impro- visational state – a continuum of not knowing, having left behind the certainty of conscious form and entered into a period of transition. Even Ruud calls this a liminal state in which 'flow' ("a psychic state where incidences follow each other in a united organic way without conscious participation") and 'void' (where old meaning is emptied out in order to create new space to be filled with new meanings") are equally vital constituents.[251]

The process of performing the dreams of the body illustrated in this book seems very similar to Paton's 'model of imagination'.[252] The creation of a performance here works with an initial conscious form into which the dancers step. They have a score, a sequence of chosen movements arising out of preparatory process. They use these movements as a starting point, first putting them on, but then intending to sink down into the movement and feel it their senses, and in their emotions, so that it comes to life inside them. They are now in a receptive, playful, 'liminal' state, involving both psyche and body, in which they are being moved, rather than directing the movement.

It is as if the formal presentation of the play creates a threshold for deepening experience. The costumes, props,

---

249   Paton, 2000.
250   Ruud,1995.
251   Paton, 2000, p. 9.
252   Paton, 2000.

lighting, music chosen, create a pattern through which the authentic body can move and dance, an interweaving of conscious choice with fluid spontaneous movement. The act of performance becomes an act of creativity, blending left and right brain faculties, in a dance between the known and the unknown.

8.2 Self-confidence, dance and visual art

The undergraduate study

Replicating Gilroy's[253] finding, experience of therapy (in this instance dance movement therapy rather than art therapy) seems to have boosted self-confidence and to have injected a sense of purpose into choreography:

> I've decided that choreography is something really personal and as long as I feel good with it that's it; to be all my life in my art, that's the whole point of art isn't it?

Confidence comes from the Latin verb confidere, which means to 'trust fully'.[254] So to have self-confidence is to place my trust fully in myself, in my own experience of my body and my soul. It is a belief in my own perception. Trust and belief happen alongside valuing and cherishing my existence, as separate body and soul and as spirit. Here it is suggested that trust in our bodies invites us into experience of emotion and imagination: the inner life or soul, and into experience of spirit, as transpersonal energy enlivening body and soul; so our bodies take on particular significance in the discussion of self-confidence.

Rogers[255] considers that an 'internal locus of evaluation' is one of the inner conditions necessary for creativity. Stern[256] writes of the development of a subjective consciousness (with the ability to independently form and evaluate ideas) as a necessary requirement for creative being. Mackinnon's[257] research on creative people, Storr's[258] theory of creativity, and more recently

---

253   Gilroy, 1989, 1992.

254   Skeat, 1978, p. 106.

255   Rogers, 1952.

256   Stern, 1985.

257   MacKinnon, 1962.

258.   Storr, 1976.

Buckroyd's[259] observations on creativity in dance all emphasise the necessity of self-confidence for creativity.

How does self-confidence impact upon creativity? I suggest it does in two significant ways. First, it feeds imagination (inspiration). It provides sensual memory with which imagination can play. It creates easeful, free-flow movement which invites emotional and imaginative experience. Second, self-confidence is a catalyst for creative action and communication (motivation). I allow my own perception and response to bear fruit in creative forms, because I value and respect my own artistic judgement (the independent evaluation named above) and because I think that my experience is worth sharing with others. I know this because I experience spirit inside me, which gives me a sense of connection to others and to the earth.

In dance movement therapy self-confidence arises out of awareness with acceptance[260] as I bring my respectful attention to my body. As I engage in a process of perceiving sensation, I acknowledge and accept my body, my emotions and my imagination and I develop trust in my own experience. Furthermore when I put my faith in my body's ability to move organically and I hand over to organic process, I open myself up to spirit as enlivening and creative energy. This is a liminal creative state[261] happening in body and mind.

Increased self-confidence was thought to be highly significant by many undergraduate dance students in helping them to develop flow of creative movement (inspiration) and to persevere with their own ideas (motivation), so that they experienced themselves as active creators.[262] Self-confidence was perceived to have developed through affirming body-rooted experience in a safe community, which promoted open, free-flow movement, sometimes used as creative resource. Dancers felt that confident experience of self had motivated them to communicate their own experience through performance.

---

259   Buckroyd, 2000.
260   Hayes, 2004.
261   Ruud, 1995.
262   Hayes, 2004.

In many instances, emotional awareness with acceptance and release, arising out of contemplative bodywork and movement,[263] was perceived to have facilitated free, self-confident movement and creativity in choreography. Students, feeling free and released from frozen emotions, felt empowered to express themselves in all their fullness in their art. In so doing they experienced themselves as creative beings.

In the following example, emotional awareness (surfacing from body awareness) seems to free the body for expanded self-expression; release of emotions through the body seems to stimulate imagery expressed through body metaphor:

> When I started to break through my blockages, I found that I really opened up in my choreography. It made quite a powerful piece on suppression and release of emotions. Very visual as well, turning images into movement.

Many dancers found that experiential dance movement therapy helped them to access and stay with their emotions. One dancer felt that she no longer needed medication for depression because she had come to terms with family tragedy. Furthermore, she was able to make this tragedy the subject of her dissertation piece, a process and performance which she described as a personal catharsis. The acceptance of her emotional pain gave her the confidence to share it in her dance. Now that she could experience herself fully, she was able to express herself fully and become creative.

> I had no confidence in choreography because there was that thing there that I couldn't let out because if I did that in my dance then everyone would see it and it was too personal. I hadn't faced it in myself so there was no way I could have aired it in front of everyone else, but now I'm going to try and go for it.

This student seems to be suggesting that her creative confidence was impeded by alienation from her emotional self; that she had to open herself up to her emotional life through her

---

263   Rockwell, 1989.

body in order to become creative. Leonard[264] asserts that creativity arises out of a person's ability to live and bear emotional pain, and come to terms with lived experience. Creativity is seen as a process of emotional awareness rather than emotional sublimation, and avoidance of emotion is considered as a pathway to sterility and self-destruction. In the above example, emotional awakening through the body certainly seems to stimulate creative process and expression.

Another dancer found that the emotions accessed through her body carried her into new expressive phrases which both she and her examiners perceived as beautiful. Sincerity gave birth to beauty[265] and gave her confidence to invest herself more in her choreography:

> Do you remember when I got upset because my Granddad had... I was really close to my Granddad. I had been think -ing about him loads and I got upset... It gave me a big phrase of material... coming out of inside. It was really quite lovely and flowing and embracing. It made me feel confident about being able to show my feelings in my movements.

Self-confidence enabled students to resist type-casting and incongruous choreographic instruction (escape from the judgment of others) and to invest themselves in their own ideas. Individuals commented on an increased sense of personal power and integrity in movement and choreography, plus increased enjoyment as well as enhanced focus during performance. Self-confidence made them feel very 'present' in their work:

> Performance can be very fake, but I've found through dance movement therapy I've been able to go on the stage and actually be me; this is me now.

The process of putting personal experience, awareness and knowledge into choreography was experienced as empowering and expansive. Many students felt that they were reaching out to others from an authentic and connected place in themselves

---

264   Leonard, 1989.
265   Trungpa, 1996.

which had both personal and transpersonal significance. This strengthened creative purpose.

The finding of enhancement of self-confidence in the undergraduate study suggests that an experiential dance movement therapy group promoting authentic movement and community may be recommended to support both the personal and creative growth of undergraduate dance students.

Enhancing self-confidence has been identified as an important goal within tertiary education generally by researchers into the mental health needs of undergraduate students[266] and it has been designated as vital for the emotional and creative growth of dance students specifically.[267]

This undergraduate study identified a tendency towards self-criticism in dance students and noted a significant change in relation to self through participation in experiential dance movement therapy:

> I expressed how I felt through movement and I can concentrate more now. Dance movement therapy has helped me focus on things, just giving time for myself to sit down and notice how I am. I feel better.

Self-acknowledgement and self-expression in experiential dance movement therapy seem to have contributed to students' well-being and focus while at university.

But what of the other side of the coin? In her study of art therapists in training, Gilroy[268] asked questions about both the stimulating and the inhibiting aspects of self-awareness through art therapy. She suggests that art therapists perceived their work to be 'more spontaneous, natural, fresher' and that they felt 'more able to play, with less self-consciousness and self-control', accepting more readily mess and chaos. Acceptance of unconscious material was experienced as stimulating; anger and violence in particular were viewed as creative resources. No

---

266   Grant, 2002.
267   Buckroyd, 2000.
268   Gilroy, 1989, 1992.

longer afraid of producing powerful images, therapists felt more able to take risks in their art. 'Letting things happen' was emphasised, and expressive, exploratory aspects of art were valued more than intellectual and aesthetic concerns. However, the counter-experience of emotional fragility due to the tendency to interpret and analyse the unconscious content of their art was also described.

Whilst above I have described how self-awareness with acceptance developed self-confidence and contributed to both creative inspiration and motivation, it also caused anxiety. Some students were aware that personal investment made them vulnerable; in relation to their assessed choreography they experienced what I have described in Chapter 2, Section 2.4 as the 'faltering' of courage to create:[269]

> I never did anything based on personal material, on emotions. It was always movement shapes etc. I never wanted to put myself up for someone else to judge.

Assessment was feared particularly by participants who felt they had put *themselves* into their work:

> I'm really happy with the way my piece is going at the moment. I don't want to be disheartened. I think it's because it's so close to me that it means so much to me. It's part of me, so if they say something about it, they say something about me. Because it's really closely connected, it scares me.

This quotation indicates how much is at stake when a student uses her own experience as creative source: when the aesthetic and the personal are hand in hand, criticism of one implies criticism of the other. Perhaps assessment needs to acknowledge more the relationship between life and art, so as to build a bridge between to two. If students are encouraged to use their own experience, they will develop their own ability to receive and design[270] and become innovators in creative practice.

---

269   May, 1975.

270   Beiswanger, 1962.

In 2003 the Performing Arts Learning and Teaching Innovation Network (PALATINE) conference questioned the rationale behind assessment in the arts and highlighted the value of formative, interactive assessment and self-assessment as important for self-confidence and creative growth. These forms of assessment, involving exploration and questioning, might be considered to be better suited to the development of self-confidence and creativity than assessment based purely on command of particular aesthetic models, which places authority with the model rather than with the student's experience.

Postgraduate and subsequent undergraduate work

Catherine, a postgraduate visual artist, whose performance of The Phoenix is in Chapter 5, writes:

> I was affected by the directness of using my own body in order to project personal metaphor. The immediacy of dance and movement to project self was something that I was fearful of. Painting onto the canvas is a similar experience, however, it is an experience I do not share; the viewer only sees the finished product.[271]

The directness of using the body to experience and communicate inner life was anxiety-provoking for this visual artist. Yet in the context of a strong 'holding circle' of community,[272] fearful feelings can be borne. Catherine's experience supports this:

> In dance, others saw the process and the shared insights helped me to understand myself better.[273]

Integration of feelings not only affects physical and mental wellbeing, it can also become a resource for imagination and transformation. As Jan Svankmajer, surrealist, artist and film-maker, writes:

> Like the alchemists of old, in my creative work I keep distilling the water of my childhood experiences,

---

271   McLelland, 2005c.
272   Chapter 2, section 2.5.
273   McLelland, 2005c.

obsessions, idiosyncracies and anxieties for there to emerge the 'heavy water' of learning necessary for the transmutation of life.[274]

Caroline Pearce-Higgins, another postgraduate visual artist, writes:

> The work was an opportunity to explore and express my feelings and experiences honestly, in a way, to unmask myself. This process was shared with others – it meant showing myself, and also receiving the messages of other people, being as open and sensitive as possible.[275]

Through body and movement exploration of conflict between suppression and expression, in the presence of affirming witnesses, Caroline realises the connection between self-confidence and creativity. She writes:

> I started my performance with the long-standing tension in myself between working in a position of responsibility as an arts administrator – drawing on my masculine-trained mind – and my desire to express myself creatively in the arts, which calls for my feminine nature. To this conflict was added the negative voice in my head that criticised me for not finding the time and the energy to keep some regular creative work going during these past seven years of my working life ('other people can'). Although I have now relinquished most of these external responsibilities, the internal issues are still current for me. As I write this, the same negative voice in me says I have no right to want, or to try, to work as an artist. This lack of confidence – which is also fear of exposing myself as I am – goes very deep and colours everything I do.[276]

Here Caroline identifies the block to her own creativity as lack of self-confidence linked to fear of self-exposure. From this point of fragile departure, she begins to let her body speak her story and provide her with a pathway to creativity. She dares to expose her

---

274   Svankmajer, (b. 1934), 1965, p. 2.

275   Pearce-Higgins, 2005a.

276   Pearce-Higgins, 2005b, pp. 1-2.

own movements, emotions and images, in the hope that they can teach her and animate her art. She touches her process of self-negation by exploring feelings of distraction and purposelessness. She finds herself crouching down, cowering away, full or fear and refusal, 'wiped out'.[277] Seeing these movements mirrored by her partner, she begins to feel compassion for herself. From this place of blackness, a rainbow begins to form and her movements become purposeful, fluid and rhythmic. Whilst such movement brings release and joy, in performance she still experiences 'an unexpected feeling of exposure and vulnerability'. She writes: 'I found it hard to believe in this sense of freedom'.[278]

Self-exposure can be a rich resource in creative process, in which we explore our cherished existence as separate entity. It requires love and compassion for self, a belief that our life and experience are intrinsically of value. It requires also a sense of connection to the lives of others; a feeling that we are part of something bigger, that our life mirrors the lives of others and that we all have value.

Self-exposure in creative process may also spring from cherished existence of self as spirit. The need for such self-exposure becomes apparent when considering Ruud's[279] and Paton's[280] model of imagination and creativity. For immersion in the organic process they describe requires the confidence to throw oneself up to chance happening, to risk defeat and failure, to find nothing or to find chaos and to trust that pattern will emerge. This is sublime self-confidence and self-exposure, which arise from experience of self as spirit, as connected to a creativity which is vast and eternal.

In her performance, Caroline experiences a tension between two forces which she defines as 'animus' (masculine self) and 'anima' (feminine self). Often her 'animus' is identified as a destructive force, wanting everything to be linear and logical,

---

277   Pearce-Higgins, 2005b, p. 2.
278   Pearce-Higgins, 2005b, p. 3.
279   Ruud, 1995.
280   Paton, 2000.

critical of lateral thought, bodily, imagistic or heartfelt experience. Yet in the process of making her play she sees a glimmer of a redefinition of 'animus':

> My purpose is to show that the animus, who is indeed like a woman's male partner, is not only irritating and destructive but is of the utmost value, and is essential for any creativeness on her part.[281]

> In a woman's world of shadows and cosmic truths the animus makes a pool of light as a focus for her eyes... [282]

Her play is a dance between 'anima' and 'animus' as potentially antagonistic opposites with no meeting-point between, but suggests the possibility of a partnership of complementary opposites. As 'animus' is redefined from 'constriction' to 'focus', the two principles may dance together, rather than fighting each other. The moments of transition between 'animus' and 'anima' are moments which may therefore be expanded in Caroline's future work.

Now Caroline continues to explore transpersonal dance movement practice, experiencing flow in body, emotion and image, releasing and activating creativity. She experiences how exposure of her own soul in the presence of non-judgemental, compassionate witnesses brings a sense of her own authentic presence, which lends vitality to her art. She now honours her soul and spirit, which strengthens her purpose, and she follows their call, heard in playful, free-flow movement, to make forms in clay.

As Caroline's self-confidence grows, she is able to explore, ever more deeply, her own story, inside her art. I suggest that it is such passionate, lived experience infused with spirit which gives art its integrity and authority. If art springs from authenticity, its message is strong; it makes people sit up and listen/behold/pay attention. If art is rooted in the soul of the artist, it reaches out to the soul of the witness. The story of one soul is connected to the story of others; spirit animates, pervades and connects us in deep kinship.

---

[281]   Claremont de Castillejo, 1990, p. 73.

[282]   Claremont de Castillejo, 1990, p. 76.

8.3: Relationship, dance and visual art

The undergraduate study

Embodiment has been identified as facilitating contact with spirit and releasing creative process in Dharma Art.[283] Through embodiment we are brought into relationship with ourselves, others, the planet and the cosmos. In embodied relationship we are able to perceive the sensations, the feelings and the images of self and others[284] as well as the rhythms and patterns of the planet and the cosmos.

Relationship was identified in the undergraduate study as one of the three major impacts of experiential dance movement therapy. The process of dance movement therapy seems to have either enhanced or intensified relationship in all cohorts. Most participants spoke about improved communication in the group as a result of relational sensitivity, whilst acknowledging the vulnerabilities which were thrown up through the process of increased intimacy (referred to as 'daunting' and 'scary').

Dancers spoke about the development of relational sensitivity:

> After the group you sort of knew whether people wanted you to be there or whether they wanted to be on their own.

The practice of non-judgemental witnessing in a non-pressurised (free from temporal and aesthetic demands) context was perceived as facilitating intersubjective intuition. In performance the kinaesthetic and emotional empathy which had developed between participants was considered to have helped the performance group to 'gel'. In choreography and performance, personal 'centering' and observation of others were perceived to have helped identify obstacles to creative flow:

---

283   Chapter 2, Section 2.2.
284   Cox & Theilgaard, 1987, p. 174.

> Being in the centre of you... and the observation, you would pick up on things, how people are, whether there are problems. I think these are new ways, which can help people to go forward on a dance level, on a performance level too.

A trusting relationship was perceived as enhancing creative communication and motivation in choreography:

> Choreography, like any form of play, needs that bond-making, you know, 'Trust me' sort of thing. You can see it through any performance that you do, there's always that element at the beginning. You have to be relaxed with the people that you work with and know where they're all coming from, to be able to give what you have to give, no holds barred.

It was felt that sensitivity alongside imagination would help a choreographer to maximise creative potential in dancers, finding contexts or movements which would allow the dancers to grow personally and creatively:

> I make space and time to observe and analyse the dancers and that helps me to imagine what I can get from the dancer as this character. It's reading body language, noticing how the dancer feels and what could be good for him to do.

Dancers' ability to empathise with their choreographer was also considered important in accessing the choreographer's intentions. One participant described her choreography as a reflection of her internal state. She felt that dancers in her piece needed to be able to empathise with her, so that her internal vision could be given accurate representation.

One participant mourned the loss of untapped creative potential due to poor relationships in the group prior to the experience of dance movement therapy:

It's too late now, you're coming to an end, there's a lot of bitchiness, favourites, non-favourites, so when you come to a session like this and you see everyone for what they are, there are so many qualities that could have been used and a lot of things that could have been learnt from other people, but you've been stuck with 'I'm working with you, I always work with you, and we work well together, but we always work in this particular way whereas it could have been all of a sudden a whole new thing set off'.

There was general lament for the unrealised creative potential, glimpsed through relationships developing in experiential dance movement therapy. Participants believed that empathy had opened up restrictive dynamics which not only influenced social interaction but also limited creative invention.

Perhaps if dance students began their relationship in an experiential dance movement therapy group, cliques would be less likely to form. Whilst misunderstandings, alienation and hostility would no doubt still surface,[285] entering into relationship in a secure open environment might offer the possibility of exploration of hostile feelings rather than indulgence in them.

Dance-making usually takes place in a group context. Choreographer and dancers work together on creating the piece. The dancers listen to the choreographer's vision and they interpret the vision through their bodies. Often dancers improvise together in order to create movement material. The need for trust, empathy and sensitivity in choreography is evident. If they are present, dancers can respond to each other authentically from their innermost experience of being. I suggest that if a group of dancers can respond to one another in this way, a dance containing both personal and transpersonal feeling and meaning results.

If creative process needs to happen in part in the realm of the unconscious,[286] that is, that it presupposes suspension of

---

285   de Maré et al., 1991.

286   Meekums, 1993; Paton, 2000; Ruud, 1995.

conscious critical faculties for part of the process, then it might be argued that artists who work together on creative projects need to have faith in the respectful witnessing of the collaborators.[287] They need to trust that their creative partners will not abuse the vulnerability involved when rational control is relinquished. If they feel that they are being judged or criticised in any way by others, they will not be willing to explore the irrational and unconscious.

Several participants described the nature of relationship in experiential dance movement therapy as 'open', 'honest' and 'direct', and when Cohort 1 subsequently created a piece together during Lea Anderson's residency, dancers and choreographer all noticed cohesiveness in the group, which was perceived as beneficial to choreographic process in both exploration and design.

Postgraduate and subsequent undergraduate work

The process of sharing body and soul with others in a safe community was perceived as significant in promoting playfulness/creativity and self-confidence in postgraduate and subsequent undergraduate work as it had been in the undergraduate study.[288] In particular, the experience of body congruence and empathy had a profound effect upon motivation for dance performance and visual art.

In expressing and witnessing embodied stories, participants gained a profound sense of connectedness to other human beings. Often from a cramped and isolating feeling of being a 'madwoman in the attic', they moved to feel their place in the human story. This sense of belonging infused their art with purpose, for communication of their own lived truth seemed now to be important because it unearthed emotions and experiences which were buried, not merely in themselves, as individuals, but in society at large.

---

287   Cottam and Sager, 2002.
288   Hayes, 2004.

The movement of energy between protagonist and audience is a tangible example of the potential for communication, empathy and healing in embodied performance. In Moira's performance, she perceives the energy of the group as all around her like a protective and generative womb. In Wynona's and Catherine's performance, the audience is energised by the growth they have witnessed and join in the dance. Likewise in Ana's performance, the audience is caught up in her rhythm, as she opens herself to the energy in her body. The energy of the dancers' bodies and in the stone is felt by the audience in Kelly's, Tracie's, Amie's and Sarah's performance. These examples suggest that the protagonist's embodied journey of healing can impact upon the audience energetically; that the body in performance can fulfil its mythic nature, stirring the energy in others.

Such stirring of energy creates the possibility of a shared 'liminal'[289] state between protagonists and audience. Body resonance and emotional and imaginative empathy create a deep level of contact with process. Everyone takes part in the play and the playing. Everyone is rapt by the emergent metaphors, and transformation is shared.

8.4 Contexts

The perceptions of the outcomes of playfulness, self-confidence and relationship arose inside the experiential dance movement therapy group in the undergraduate study.[290] They were also experienced in the postgraduate and subsequent undergraduate context of transpersonal dance movement practice in a process and performance community.

In Chapter 2, Section 2.5, the concept of the 'holding circle' of the group was defined as 'a visual image for a united, compassionate presence, which launches the protagonists in their venture to bear or suffer their truth'. The 'holding circle' affirms the energy in the body, the passion of the emotions, the forms of the imagination in each individual. Body, emotion and

---

289   Ruud, 1995.
290   Hayes, 2004.

imagination are given deep respect. The circle lets them be and lets them out. For, in the circle, they are respected as the essence of the person's life and the life of the community too. They are perceived as expressions of bodyspirit.

In postgraduate and subsequent undergraduate work, compassionate presence was perceived to have been created from non-judgemental witnessing of authentic movement, and in the undergraduate study it was perceived to have evolved through the group's willingness to accept all members or to have been threatened by the group's tendency to criticise. For further elaboration of the breaking-down of trust, please refer to Chapter 7 of the undergraduate study.[291]

In the undergraduate study, the positive outcomes (playfulness, self-confidence and relationship) of experiential dance movement therapy were attributed to play, movement metaphor, acceptance and safety. These components are all present in transpersonal dance movement practice, where participants are encouraged to allow their bodies to play, expressing feeling and image through movement, which is received with respect in empathic witnessing.

I suggest that the 'holding circle' may be transferred as a supportive concept to dance education and training. Students of dance frequently make themselves vulnerable as they expose their bodies, their hearts and their minds to their fellows and to their teachers. In developing a compassionate context, we are facilitating the emergence of creativity in the individual and in the community.

---

[291]   Hayes, 2004.

Chapter 9

Therapy

This chapter examines the relevance of transpersonal dance movement practice for the 'talking therapies'. Many of the students on the postgraduate courses, from which the performances in this book derive, were qualified experienced counsellors, psychotherapists or psychoanalysts. They referred to 'the transformational experience' of transpersonal dance movement practice and perceived that it had enriched their practice of verbal counselling, psychotherapy or psychoanalysis.

I will use the terms counsellor, psychotherapist and psychoanalyst with reference to specific contributions to the study. Elsewhere I will use the generic terms practitioner, therapist and therapy to cover all therapeutic practice here researched. As in Chapter 2 I use the term soulseeker for the person in therapy, as someone who is searching to embody their inner experience; this person is not perceived as ill, but as trying to return to the blueprint of growth and development which is a birthright. Sometimes the term client is used for convenience, as it is commonly used in contemporary therapeutic practice where it is intended to empower through its association with choice and employment of service. Of course it reflects the capitalist structure of Western culture, and does not express transpersonal quality in the therapeutic relationship.

The terms used to focus the discussion of practitioners' response to and application of transpersonal dance movement practice are congruence and empathy. These terms come from person-centred practice, but are, I suggest, relevant to all approaches to therapeutic process. In contemporary therapeutic practice, authentic contact in the therapeutic relationship is valued in all approaches.[292]

---

292   Clarkson, 1995; Kahn, 1997.

Many practitioners in this study referred to a change from estrangement to belonging in their body as sacred home:

> I was quite profoundly affected by the movement-based work. It brought me into a 'gut' (rather than simply cerebral) awareness of the body as sacred... of the body as having its own integrity. I had never previously trusted or respected or loved my body. I had not paid much attention to it. I had valued my senses – sight, hearing, touch, taste, smell – but I thought of myself as a clumsy mover and an incompetent dancer. It was very exciting for me to discover that my body had something of its own to say, which only happened when I silenced my will, my planning mind, my busy intentions, my desire for control. I had previously learned how to still my body (e.g. in meditation). I had not learned how to let it move naturally, i.e. according to its own nature. I discovered that my body is actually quite graceful. I can move in ways that surprise me. I do consciously experience myself, now (most of the time – there are lapses!) as embodied: that is I notice my delight in subtle sensing and moving. I am lighter. I was stunned when someone said to me recently, "You know how to live in your own body". This was definitely not the case before I participated in the movement-based work.

This experience of the body dancing its own dance and having its own integrity reflects the rationale of the work described in this book. The body here is seen as part of nature, its frame permitting movement in four directions, facilitating opening up and expansion, closing and contraction, propulsion through space and relationship. Organic movement through the frame of the body is cultivated through a process of silent sensing and subsequent expression of energetic rhythm. The underlying rationale behind this work is that our form permits a beautiful and graceful expression and release of energy as do all organic forms on earth. Through organic movement our bodies help us to be aware of our relationship to our planet. When we let the energy all around us, flow through us, we become part of the dance of spirit.

Pinkola Estes[293] writes of the emotional expression of skin and moving body. She describes the body as a 'multi-lingual being',[294] a concept akin to Hanna's[295] definition of 'soma' home to all of human experience, physical, emotional, mental. The body's ability to perceive the world and to creatively express emotional and mental response is remarkable. Dance and movement can show directly to a witness our many ways of experiencing the world, without one word being spoken.

Practitioners in this study were surprised at the depth of contact found in the witnessing relationship of Authentic Movement. Witnesses frequently perceived feelings and images in the mover which mirrored the mover's experience. Deep connection to self and others was a commonly perceived effect of movement process, one which was carried away and into the therapy room with clients. As one psychoanalyst comments:

> I feel so refreshed in my empathy. Even as I sit in my consulting room and my patient sits almost opposite, I sense the movements and the currents of feeling between us. My work has been (re)-embodied and for that I feel grateful.

McNiff [296] writes:

> The successes and failures of the therapy work we do are closely connected to energetic qualities that we have yet to even acknowledge. We need to study what this energy does: how it can be cultivated, how it circulates through people and environments, how it might be described and assessed, what effects it has upon people, and how it finds its way to areas in need of transformation.[297]

---

293   Pinkola Estes, 1992.

294   Pinkola Estes, 1992, p. 200.

295   Hanna, 1970.

296   McNiff, 2004.

297   McNiff, 2004, p. 212.

The movement-based work described in this book and the performances arising out of it have shown how immersion in our bodies can tap into a stream of animating energy. As the mind makes way for physical experiencing, the body is released into an organic flow of energy. By focusing our minds upon this, we become aware of this flow of energy inside us and around us. Sensitive contemplation and dynamic expression of body-felt experience may therefore connect us to spirit in self and others, facilitating organic process, evolution and completion, bringing healing and transformation. This enriches life and art, and is particularly significant for therapeutic process.

Attunement with energy in authentic movement may be linked to the concept of congruence[298] in counselling and psychotherapy, which originated in the work of the humanistic psychologist and pioneer of the person-centred approach to counselling and psychotherapy, Carl Rogers. It is defined as a state in which a person is fully and deeply themselves with awareness.[299] Whilst Rogers himself does not dwell on the body as source of congruence, Gendlin,[300] a contemporary of Rogers, devotes a book to the practice of 'focussing': an attentiveness to the body, as guide in freely experiencing emotion. The body as place of personal growth and development is currently receiving much more attention in humanistic and person-centred practice.[301]

The data for this chapter are postgraduate practitioners' perceptions of transpersonal dance and movement practice and of its relevance for verbal counselling, psychotherapy and psychoanalysis. Perceptions are discussed anonymously under the heading 'congruence and empathy'. These concepts have been chosen as best representing the comments from 30 questionnaires. The discussion below shows how congruence and empathy intertwine, as self-awareness opens up channels of perception and communication.

---

298   Natiello, 2001; Pearmain, 2001; Wyatt, 2001.
299   Rogers, [1902-1987], 1957.
300   Gendlin, 1981.
301   Cooper, 2001.

There were two questions asked: 1. Were you affected by the movement-based work? If so, how? 2. Has the movement-based work had any effect upon your client work? If so, how? As in the undergraduate study of student dancers in higher education,[302] this is a piece of qualitative research in which participants' perceptions have been subjectively embraced and creatively interpreted and organised by the researcher. Subjectivity and creativity are acknowledged and valued as sources of knowledge and as insightful avenues of communication.[303] It was specifically the willingness to be involved in the movement processes and performances of the research participants which opened me up, as researcher, to their experience. Through embodied relationship I was able, like others in the 'holding circle' of the process, performance and research group, to perceive the subsequently confirmed depth experience of the mover, and to respond holistically to the personal and the archetypal stories.

This research into the experience of the body was organic in its approach.[304] Transpersonal dance movement practice created a space for organic movement which could be contemplated with respect and awe. The body's movement was researched with appreciation and enjoyment. Feelings and images were accepted and explored with eagerness and surprise. The happenings in the body and the connections to spirit were recorded with attention and devotion. It is hoped that the findings here may be compared and contrasted with the findings from other research into transpersonal therapeutic process.

Payne[305] has examined the experience of trainee verbal counsellors and therapists in personal development groups during their training. She has also researched the experience of trainee dance movement therapists in an experiential dance movement therapy group.[306] Like Gilroy,[307] in the field of art

---

302   Hayes, 2004

303   Anderson, 1998; Braud and Anderson, 1998; Moustakas, 1981, 1990.

304   Clements, Ettling, Jenett, Shields, 1998.

305   Payne, 1999, 2001.

306   Payne, 1996.

307   Gilroy, 1989, 1992.

therapy, Payne found that whilst the experience was one of enhancing congruence, this sometimes brought with it an increased sense of vulnerability, which was sometimes disabling for trainee therapists in practice placements, when the ability to hold another's pain and fracture was essential.

It may be argued that personal process work is a necessary foundation for work as a therapist, and must not be excluded from therapy training, on the basis that therapist congruence will be superficial unless deep connection with subjective internal process is cultivated. If the experience of self is superficial, then it will never be more than a shaky resource upon which to practise therapy. Intuitive responding will not be possible, for the ground of self, from which intuition springs, has not been tilled. Payne's[308] research findings suggest that personal process work needs to happen *before* the trainee ventures into practice.

In the research described in this book, the population was different. The movement-based work was part of continuing professional development for established practitioners. These people had undertaken years of personal therapy and professional training and were established advanced practitioners in their field. The expectation was that these professionals would be able to continue to hold others in their professional practice whilst exploring personal process through movement.

Still the movement-based work brought them into a different experience of their stories, a physical experience, and this physical understanding was both turbulent and transformative. During this period of personal exploration, most of the practitioners continued to hold the process work of others because they were practised at containing their own process. Whilst it has been suggested that personal process work is a necessary foundation for work as a therapist, it is also a continual process in which the therapist is constantly engaging with experience, to nurture personal congruence. Perhaps with past experience of personal process work, the therapist is better equipped to engage with it whilst practising, and perhaps also

---

308   Payne, 1996.

there will be times when the therapist needs to take a break from holding others so that she too can give full respect to her inner life for the sake of her own creativity as a person and as a therapist.

9.1: Congruence and empathy

Congruence has been defined above as being truly and deeply oneself with awareness. Like Gendlin,[309] I believe that emotional presence with awareness may be developed through attention to the body and the body's movement. Also I believe, like Cox and Theilgaard,[310] that imaginative presence with awareness may be promoted through attention to the body and the body's movement. Finally, I have argued in Part 1 that spiritual presence with awareness may be cultivated through transpersonal dance movement practice.

In this study of practitioners' response to transpersonal dance movement practice, sensation was perceived as threshold to spirit. It was as if the awakening of the body set spirit free in the body and facilitated a corresponding awakening of emotion and imagination. This new experience of body, spirit, emotion and imagination in self created receptivity to corresponding aspects of experience in others, and facilitated empathic relationship. As one counsellor writes:

> I have a greater awareness of my untapped potential ...a spiritual dimension I was not aware of... I feel I had some access/insight into this as a result of the movement work. This has brought personal growth/development which has opened me up – an opening up to experience – for myself and in my work with others: embracing experience rather than being shut/closed to experience.

The link between congruence and empathy is clearly present in this example. In becoming more sensitised and open to her own spiritual creative potential, the counsellor feels more capable of embracing the potential of her clients. She feels herself to be 'opened up to experience', able to let more in, more

---

309   Gendlin, 1981.
310   Cox and Theilgaard, 1987 p. 174.

receptive to the unfamiliar. This must certainly be helpful to therapeutic process, for the welcoming of all experience, no matter what, by the therapist, allows the client to bring all of her experience, conscious and unconscious, into the therapy room. It invites the soulseeker to be who she is in all her fullness. Such acceptance and encouragement of all that we are and may be honours our human potential and heals any wounds caused by oppression of spirit.

The stir of potential in self and community is noticed by other practitioners:

> The coming together of movement, feeling, thought and a sense of community was very moving – electrifying even. All aspects of my awareness were brought into life-enhancing energy, and there was a stir in what had previously lain still and silent.

It is as if something new is being brought into life which invigorates the individual and fosters connection between members of the group.

A counsellor writes:

> In the movement-based work I felt deeply affirmed and respected in my being just so. I could be there wholly as myself, taking away the defensive behaviours, at least some layers, and experiencing how it is to show what's underneath.

> I am more at one with myself in my communications with clients; I can tolerate more fears and uncertainty rather than insisting on rigid structure.

In this example, affirmation and respect are named as the qualities present in the group which promote congruence. These qualities were found to be highly significant in the study of student dancers' experience in an experiential dance movement therapy group[311] in developing playfulness, self-confidence and relationship. Here, in this study of practitioners' experience of

---

311   Hayes, 2004.

transpersonal dance movement practice, respect and non-judgemental witnessing are perceived as facilitating self-acceptance and self-expression in the group, as well as congruence in professional practice. Trust in self ripples outwards as trust in process in both transpersonal dance movement practice and professional work: fear and uncertainty can be tolerated, without the compulsion to make superficial order. Sinking down into the physical experience of being brings with it inner certainty and self-respect which stands firm in situations of uncertainty, and helps us as practitioners to be present with the uncertainty of process.

In transpersonal dance movement practice we learn to let ourselves be as we are, and we give ourselves time to sense our physical and psychic reality before we share it with others. Self-knowledge and self-respect feed our capacity to respect others, to give them time to sense and express how they are. We no longer wish or usher others to feel something other than authentic sensation and emotion in that moment. We are unhurried, we wait for them to tell their story. Such respectful attention facilitates the emergence of authentic experience in therapy, and so encourages spirit to enliven and propel human life. A counsellor describes a feeling of 'stillness' in relationship:

> I am much stiller than before when clients are talking of distressing things.

There are numerous examples of practitioners linking physical with emotional and transpersonal awareness:

> I was very closed physically, which mirrored the effects of past trauma. The work enabled me for the first time to fill my personal space and spread my arms out... liberating physically and emotionally and more so, spiritually.

> It put me in touch with deep aspects of my personality, especially the power of the animus and shadow. It helped me to feel more integrated.

The movement-based work was both deepening and freeing. The culminating performance allowed me to come more to terms with childhood and generational loss and trauma.

The movement was extremely beneficial to me. It enabled me to connect with my deepest pain, to express it authentically and to release it.
Through this I felt liberated and cleansed.

Enhancement of congruence and empathy in professional practice is a common finding:

This has affected my work because I am so changed.

I realised how tense my body felt; now I am more aware of my physical and feeling response to clients.

If I receive the message from my clients that bodywork may help expression/contact/open up blocks, then I will create a safe place for them to be in their bodies and find out where and how they need to be.

I have seen more connection between my clients' movement and their state of mind.

It was a reminder that it is the body that is often the key to contacting long-held trauma and tensions, enabling their release.

These quotations represent the perceptions of many others. Clearly, giving the body permission to move freely brought with it identification and release of blocked energy in physical, emotional and imaginative channels of experience. It established a connection with inner experience, which was both vital and revitalising. The words liberation, release and integration are used to describe an energising process of self-acceptance and self-expression, which brings with it connection to others in therapy.

In contrast, a very different experience, one of physical awkwardness, is also appreciated by one counsellor for the insight it gave her into some of her clients' stories:

> I felt very tight and restricted, and envied other group members who appeared more relaxed.

> I have a heightened awareness of client body language and inhibited movement. My experience – albeit personally negative – has helped me become instinctively empathic towards those who likewise feel uncomfortable in strange new relationships or settings.

Another psychotherapist acknowledges that sensing his moving body has put him in touch with his experience of fear, which helps him to connect with fear in other people.

In one instance, embodiment helped the psychotherapist to identify her need to withdraw from professional practice, to attend to her own need for self-healing:

> I connected to the physical depletion/exhaustion of my ailing body, soul, spirit, and my desperate need for love, stillness and peace. At the same time I became aware of my need/desire to connect with the group/community and to feel at one with humanity/god. I felt empowered to seek ways and means to meet my needs for stillness, peace and community in my life within and without.

> Later, I attended in a highly vulnerable/sensitive state of being, following a bereavement of an intimate other. I was thus concerned with protecting myself, listening/monitoring my own voice/process and thus erecting necessary boundaries. I connected to my own separateness/ individuality through embodying the parameters/strength of my body. I felt empowered to seek ways and means to listen to and express my own voice, give myself space, protect myself from outside influences, erect boundaries, set limits in my life within and without and to seek out the necessary medical support.

> I am currently not working professionally. The movement-based work helped me to recognise that I needed time out from the world/therapeutic work in order to heal myself and to learn to better take care of myself.

In this instance the process of letting her body speak enabled this psychotherapist to appreciate her physical, emotional and mental depletion and to honour it with self-protecting action in life and work. Such ethical reflection and action safeguards the individual and the profession. Others who had felt replenished by transpersonal dance movement practice decided to continue practising in privately facilitated groups, as a tool for 'self-nurturing, therapeutic investigation – developing an inner witness'.

Many reflections make the link between freedom of movement and freedom of imagination. It is as if the release of energy through movement occurs concurrently with the release of imagination.[312] Here is one example, where external props are also used to enhance symbolic experience:

> Combining free movement with specific items e.g. scarves and material, was particularly powerful. The individual items provided an abstract focus and combined with the freedom to move around in any desired way, something happened that surprised me. The scarves and material formed a rectangle and in that moment I was dancing round the coffin of my dead partner. This sounds really morbid and perhaps over-sensational, but it was a pleasant feeling because I never went to the funeral.

Many participants were profoundly affected by the imagery which flowed into their minds when they began to move. Sometimes images came with movement and props as in the above example, sometimes it emerged in authentic movement with eyes closed. Sometimes imagery was localised, linked to situations from an individual's past, and sometimes it was perceived as archetypal or mythic: speaking of humanity.

---

312   Halprin, 1995; Halprin, 2003.

However the images were received or interpreted, participants felt more deeply connected to their imagination, and this became a valued resource in their professional practice, linking them to their own and to their clients' emotions. The body metaphor of rolling on the floor as a lion cub amidst other lion cubs, belly full of milk, connected a counsellor to her physical and emotional need to be a part of a family where physical and emotional needs are listened to. This in turn connected her to her clients' needs for physical and emotional sustenance.

Generally, the practitioners in this study perceived themselves to be much more attuned to their bodies' perceptions and responses in the therapeutic relationship as a result of engagement with transpersonal dance movement practice, and they became much more particularly attentive to the body expression of their clients:

> I can listen better to my body's signals, felt-senses.

> I find myself taking much more interest in the way people enter and leave a room, whether and how they fidget, what areas of their body they touch most, etc.

They linked motion with emotion in the therapeutic relationship:

> I sense the movements and currents of feeling between us.

They found images of soul through embodied imagination:

> The pain of becoming more conscious is the struggle of the soul as it rolls in the mud of experience.

These perceptions of enhancement of sensitivity in therapeutic relationship resulting from transpersonal dance movement practice suggest that such practice is relevant to the continuing professional development of practice in the 'talking therapies'. An appreciation of the body and the body's movement has facilitated professional growth in the verbal practitioners in this study. A heightened awareness of the perceptual and expressive body has become a tool in the verbal therapeutic relationship outside of the dance studio where transpersonal dance and movement first took place.

In the previous chapter I have proposed the inclusion of experiential dance movement therapy, transpersonal dance movement practice and Authentic Movement in dance education and training, as resources for enhancing creativity in dance. Here I conclude, like Payne,[313] with a recommendation for their use in the continuing professional development of verbal counsellors, psychotherapists and psychoanalysts.

---

[313]   Payne, 2006.

Chapter 10

A farewell

The experience of embodiment is one which is difficult to describe in words. For we often perceive and express much more through our bodies than we can tell about with words. One student writes:

> Part of my own difficulty with academia is its necessity to explain or put words on experiences. I wonder how much we gain and how much we lose.

This has been my attempt to put into words the amazing embodied experiences and performances which I have witnessed. I hope that with words I have been faithful to the embodied performances, whilst recognising that I have created new forms, based on originals. I trust that my faithful witnessing of the performances and the processes which preceded them, gave me authority to recreate them and to comment upon them. The plays have been read and edited by the protagonists and they are satisfied that they are an accurate representation of their experience.

The plays of animation and compassion have shown how the body puts us in contact with spirit inside and around us. They have shown how the body connects us to our emotions: to our deepest longings, needs, fears and hopes. They have shown too how the moving body unites with imagination to make vivid embodied images, with local, archetypal and mythic significance. In conclusion, they have shown how the body can be home to spirit, and how spirit enlivens both body and soul.

A dancer writes:

> The movement-based work gave me a feeling of release, and of connecting with a power beyond myself.

> It made me feel cleansed and happy to be alive. The world became a wonderful place and the people in the room became beautiful. It permitted a flowing of energy.

It is such 'flowing of energy' which permits growth, new birth, opening to experience, awakening, unfolding. Cox and Theilgaard describe The Aeolian Mode of therapy, which welcomes the birth of images as spontaneous healing forms of imagination. The emergence of new forms/images is described as 'poeisis': a 'threshhold occasion',[314] arising in 'the momentum of the moment'.[315] I seize on the word 'momentum' for it suggests an energetic moment. The body as sensory perceiver and receiver of energy may be the threshhold for 'poeisis', an instrument of imagination. I suggest that the channelling of spirit through the metaphoric body unites body, spirit, emotion and imagination, and fulfills the creative potential of bodyspirit.

These plays of animation and compassion are powerful examples of the ability of the human body to receive and creatively express spirit. In his essay 'The spiritual problem of modern man'[316] Jung writes:

> If we can reconcile ourselves with the mysterious truth that spirit is the living body seen from within, and the body the outer manifestation of the living spirit – the two being really one – then we can understand why it is that the attempt to transcend the present level of consciousness must give its due to the body.

In performing the dreams of our bodies we embrace and express spirit, leaping across the threshold between the invisible and the visible. Our bodies form an arc of colour, intense, vibrant and fleeting; like a rainbow, vital for a moment, then dissolving into invisibility again. Through our bodies we catch a glimpse of a beauty to which we are bound because it is held in the longing of our hearts.

---

314   Cox and Theilgaard, 1987, p. 23.
315   Cox and Theilgaard, 1987, p. 25.
316   Jung, 1933, pp. 253-254.

REFERENCES

Adler J (1972) Integrity of Body and Psyche: Some Notes on Work in Progress. *Proceedings of the Seventh Annual Conference of the American Dance Therapy Association*, 42-53.

Adler J (1996) *Arching Backward*. US: Inner Traditions International.

Adler J (1999) Body and Soul. In Pallaro P (ed) (1999) *Authentic Movement: Essays by Mary Starks Whitehouse, Janet Adler and Joan Chodorow*. London: Jessica Kingsley Publishers.

Adler J (2002) *Offering from the Conscious Body*. Vermont: Inner Traditions.

Anderson R (1998) Intuitive inquiry: a transpersonal approach. In Braud W, Anderson R (eds) (1998) *Transpersonal Research Methods for the Social Sciences: Honoring Human Experience*. London: Sage.

Bachelard G (1990) (Trans. Kenneth Haltman). *Fragments of a Poetics of Fire*. Dallas, TX: Dallas Institute of Humanities and Culture

Bartal L, Ne'eman N (1993) *The Metaphoric Body. Guide to Expressive Therapy through Images and Archetypes*. London: Jessica Kingsley Publishers.

Beiswanger G (1962) Chance and design in choreography. In Nadel MH, Nadel Miller C (eds) (1978) *The Dance Experience*. New York, NY: Universe Books.

Blom L, Chaplin, L (2000) *The Moment of Movement*. London: Dance Books.

Bosnak R (1998) *A Little Course in Dreams*. Boston, MA: Shambhala Publications.

Boxhall M (2005) Breath of Life. www.stillness.co.uk

Braud W, Anderson R (eds) (1998) *Transpersonal Research Methods for the Social Sciences: Honoring Human Experience*. London: Sage.

Buckroyd J (2000) *The Student Dancer: Emotional Aspects of the Teaching and Learning of Dance*. London: Dance Books.

Burnford H, Barnham K (eds) (1997) *My Treasury of Fairy Tales*. Godalming, Surrey: Zigzag Publishing.

Cameron R (2001) In the Space Between. In Wyatt G, Sanders P (eds) (2001) *Contact and Perception*. Ross-on-Wye: PCCS Books.

Cattanach A (1995) Drama and Play Therapy with Young Children. *The Arts in Psychotherapy*, 22 (3), 223-228.

Cheney S (ed) (1977) *The Art of Dance*. New York, NY: Theatre Arts.

Chodorow J (1991) *Dance Therapy and Depth Psychology*. The Moving Imagination. London: Routledge.

Chodorow J (2006) The archetypal affect system: from the source (primordial self) to the goal (realised self). Work in progress.

Claremont de Castillejo I (1990) *Knowing Woman: A Feminine Psychology*. Boston, MA: Shambhala Publications.

Clarkson P (1995) *The Therapeutic Relationship*. London: Whurr Publishers.

Clements J, Ettling D, Jenett D, Shields L (1998) Organic research: feminine spirituality meets transpersonal research. In Braud W, Anderson R (eds) (1998) *Transpersonal research methods for the Social Sciences: Honoring Human Experience*. London: Sage.

Cooper JC (1998) *An Illustrated Encyclopaedia of Traditional Symbols*. London: Thames & Hudson.

Cooper M (2001) Embodied empathy. In Haugh S, Merry T (eds) (2001) *Empathy*. Ross-on-Wye: PCCS Books.

Cottam M, Sager P (2002) Following the Arc: An Ongoing Dialogue about Performance and Authentic Movement. *Contact Quarterly*, Summer/ Fall.

Cox M, Theilgaard A (1987) *Mutative Metaphors in Psychotherapy: The Aeolian Mode*. London: Tavistock.

Cozolino L (2002) *The Neuroscience of Psychotherapy: Building and Rebuilding the Human Brain*. London: WW Norton & Company.

Dadd M (2005) Embodying myth supporting paper. Unpublished MA paper. University of Chichester.

Dadd M (2007) Becoming wholehearted: using performance-based authentic movement and creative arts therapy to heal the wounds of trauma from childhood abandonment. Unpublished MA dissertation. University of Chichester

Dekker K (1996) Why oblique and why Jung? In Pearson J (ed) (1996) *Discovering the Self Through Drama and Movement: The Sesame Approach*. London: Jessica Kingsley Publishers.

Dunn D (1999) Making dances. In Marranca B, Dasgupta G (eds) (1999) *Conversations on Art and Performance*. Baltimore, MD: Johns Hopkins University Press.

de Mare P, Piper R, Thompson S (1991) *Koinonia: From Hate, Through Dialogue, To Culture in the Large Group*. London: Karnac Books.

Gendlin ET(1981) *Focusing*. New York: Bamtam.

Gilroy A (1989) On occasionally being able to paint. *Inscape*, Spring.

Gilroy A (1992) Art therapists and their art. A study of occupational choice and career development, from the origins of an interest in art to occasionally being able to paint. Unpublished PhD, University of Sussex, Brighton, UK.

Grant A (2002) Identifying students' concerns: taking a whole institutional approach. In Stanley N, Manthorpe J (eds) (2002) *Students' Mental Health Needs*. London: Jessica Kingsley Publishers.

Gordon R (1975) The creative process: self-expression and self-transcendence. In Jennings S (ed) (1975) *Creative Therapy*. London: Pitman.

Halprin A (1995) *Moving Toward Life*. Hanover, NH: Wesleyan University Press.

Halprin A (2000) *Dance as a Healing Art: Returning to Health With Movement and Imagery*. Mendecino, CA: LifeRhythm.

Halprin D (2003) *The Expressive Body in Life, Art and Therapy*. London: Jessica Kingsley Publishers.

Hanna T (1970) *Bodies in Revolt*. New York, NY: Holt, Rinehart & Winston.

Harpur P (2002) *The Philosopher's Secret Fire*. A History of the Imagination. London: Penguin.

Harris J (2001) *Jung and Yoga: The Psyche-Body Connection*. Toronto: Inner City Books.

Hartley L (2004) *Somatic Psychology: Body, Mind and Meaning*. London: Whurr Publications.

Hayes J (1990) *All my life*. Unpublished poem.

Hayes J (2004) The experience of student dancers in higher education in a dance movement therapy group, with reference to choreography and performance. Unpublished PhD, University of Hertfordshire.

Hillman J (1975) Revisioning Psychology. New York NY: Harper Collins Publishers Inc.

Hillman J (1992) The practice of beauty. *Sphinx: A Journal for Archetypal Psychology and the Arts*, 4. London: London Convivium for Archetypal Studies.

Hillman J (1996) *Healing Fiction*. Woodstock, CT.: Spring Publications.

Hillman, J. (1997) *The Thought of the Heart and the Soul of the World*. Woodstock, CT.: Spring Publications.

Holmes K (2005) Reflections on process and performance. Unpublished BA paper. University of Chichester.

Houston G (1993) *Being and Belonging – Group, Intergroup and Gestalt*. Chichester: John Wiley & Sons.

Houston J (1987) *The Search for the Beloved: Journeys in Mythology and Sacred Psychology*. New York, NY: Tarcher Putnam.

Houston J (1996) *A Mythic Life*. London: Harper Collins.

Jennings S (ed) (1975) *Creative Therapy*. London: Pitman.

Jones P (1996) *Drama as Therapy: Theatre as Living*. London: Routledge.

Jung CG (1933) *Modern Man in Search of a Soul*. London: Routledge.

Jung CG (1953-1979) *The Collected Works. (Bollingen Series XX)*, Princeton: Princeton University Press.

Kahn M (1997) *Between Therapist and Client: The New Relationship*. New York, NY: W.H. Freeman & Company.

Kaspar W (2005) Embodying myth supporting paper. Unpublished MA paper. University of Chichester.

Kuhlewind G (1988) *From Normal to Healthy: Paths to Liberation of Consciousness*. MA: Lindisfarne Press.

Kurtz R (1990) *Body-Centred Psychotherapy: The Hakomi Method*. Mendecino, CA: LifeRhythm.

Langer SK (1953) *Feeling and Form*. London: Routledge.

Leonard L (1989) *Witness to the Fire: Creativity and the Veil of Addiction*. Boston, MA: Shambhala Publications.

Lawrence DH (1982) Snake. In Roberts M (ed) (1982) *The Faber Book of Modern Verse* (fourth edition). London: Faber and Faber Ltd.

Levine P (1997) Waking the Tiger, Healing Trauma. Berkeley, CA: North Atlantic Books.

Levy F (1988) *Dance Movement Therapy: A Healing Art*. Virginia, USA: The American Alliance for Health, Physical education, Recreation and Dance.

Levy F (1995) (ed) *Dance and Other Expressive Arts Therapies*. London: Routledge.

Liebowitz G (1992) Individual dance movement therapy in an in-patient psychiatric setting. In Payne H (ed) (1992) *Dance Movement Therapy: Theory and Practice*. London: Routledge.

Mackinnon DW (1962) What makes a person creative? In Nadel MH, Nadel Miller C (eds) (1978) *The Dance Experience*. New York, NY: Universe Books.

Macy J (1991) *World as Lover, World as Self*. Berkeley, CA.: Parallax Press.

Martin J (1972) *The Modern Dance*. Originally published in 1933. New York, NY: Dance Horizons.

Maslow AH (1976) *The Further Reaches of Human Nature*. London: Penguin.

Masterman T (2005) Reflections on process and performance. Unpublished BA paper. University of Chichester.

May R (1975) *The Courage to Create*. London: Collins.
McTaggart C (2007) Body and Soul. Unpublished Poem.

McLelland C (2005a) Live performance recorded on video. Author's private archive.

McLelland C (2005b) Embodying myth supporting paper. Unpublished MA paper. University of Chichester.

McLelland C (2005c) Research questionnaire. Author's databank.

McNiff S (1992) *Art as Medicine: Creating a Therapy of the Imagination*. Boston, MA: Shambhala Publications.

McNiff S (2004) *Art Heals: How Creativity Cures the Soul*. Boston, MA: Shambhala Publications.

Meekums B (1993) Research as an act of creation. In Payne H (ed) (1993) *Handbook of Inquiry in the Arts Therapies: One River Many Currents*. London: Jessica Kingsley Publishers.

Meekums B (1998) Recovery from child sexual abuse trauma within an arts therapies programme for women. Unpublished PhD, Faculty of Education, University of Manchester, Manchester, UK.

Meekums B (2002) *Dance Movement Therapy*. London: Sage.

Mindell A (1995) Moving the Dreambody. *Contact Quarterly*, Winter/ Spring, 56-62.

Mirabai (2002) In my travels I spent time with a great yogi. In Ladinsky D (ed) (2002). Love Poems From God. New York, NY: Penguin Group.

Moore T (1992) Care of the Soul. A Guide for Cultivating Depth and Sacredness in Everyday Life. New York NY: Harper Collins Publishers Inc.

Moustakas C (1981) Heuristic research. In Reason P, Rowan J (eds) *Human Inquiry: A Sourcebook for New Paradigm Research*. Chichester: John Wiley & Sons.

Moustakas C (1990) *Heuristic Research: Design, Methodology and Applications*. Newbury Park, CA: Sage.

Musicant S (1994) Authentic Movement and Dance Therapy. *American Journal of Dance Therapy*, 16 (2): 91-106.

Musicant S (2001) Authentic Movement: clinical considerations. *American Journal of Dance Therapy*, 23 (1): 17-26.

Nadel MH, Nadel Miller C (eds) (1978) *The Dance Experience*. New York, NY: Universe Books.

Natiello P (2001) *The Person-Centred Approach: A Passionate Presence*. Ross-on-Wye: PCCS Books.

O'Donohue J (1998) *Eternal Echoes: Exploring our Hunger to Belong*. London: Bantam.

O'Donohue J (1999) *Anam Cara: Spiritual Wisdom from the Celtic World*. London: Bantam.

Ohlson, C (2004) Analysis of process. Unpublished BA paper. University of Chichester.

Pallaro P (ed) (1999) *Authentic Movement: Essays by Mary Starks Whitehouse, Janet Adler and Joan Chodorow*. London: Jessica Kingley Publishers.

Paton R (2000) Unpublished research paper presented at the annual conference of the International Society for Music Education Research, Exeter University, UK.

Payne HL (1992) *Dance Movement Therapy: Theory and Practice*. London: Routledge.

Payne HL (1996) The experience of a dance movement therapy group in training. Unpublished PhD, University of London, London, UK.

Payne HL (1999) Personal development groups in the training of counsellors and therapists: a review of the research. *European Journal of Psychotherapy, Counselling and Health*, 2(1): 55-68.

Payne HL (2001) Student experiences in a personal development group: the question of safety. *European Journal of Psychotherapy, Counselling and Health*, 4(2): 267-292.

Payne HL (2006) The body as container and expresser: Authentic Movement groups in the development of wellbeing in our bodymindspirit. In Corrigall J, Payne H, Wilkinson H (eds) (2006) *About a Body: Working with the Embodied Mind in Psychotherapy*.

Pearce-Higgins C (2005a) Research questionnaire. Author's databank.

Pearce-Higgins C (2005b) Embodying myth supporting paper. Unpublished MA paper. University of Chichester.

Pearmain R (2001) *The Heart of Listening: Attentional Qualities in Psychotherapy*. London: Continuum.

Pearson J (ed) (1996) *Discovering the Self through Drama and Movemen: The Sesame Approach*. London: Jessica Kingsley Publishers.

Pinkola Estes C (1992) *Women Who Run With the Wolves: Contacting the Power of the Wild Woman*. London: Rider.

Powlesland A (2005) Reflections on process and performance. Unpublished BA paper. University of Chichester.

Reed S (2005) Reflections on process and performance. Unpublished BA paper. University of Chichester.

Reich W (1933) *Character Analysis*. New York, NY: Farrar, Strauss & Giroux.

Rezende-Miggin A (2005) Embodying myth supporting paper. Unpublished MA paper. University of Chichester.

Rilke RM (1902) Evening. In Mitchell S (ed, trans) (1995) *Ahead of All Parting: The Selected Poetry and Prose of Rainer Maria Rilke*. New York, NY: Random House Inc.

Rilke RM (1911-1920) Turning point. In Mitchell S (ed, trans) (1995) *Ahead of All Parting: The Selected Poetry and Prose of Rainer Maria Rilke.* New York, NY: Random House Inc.

Rockwell IN (1989) Dance: Creative Process from a Contemplative Point of View. In: *Dance: Current Selected Research.* New York: AMS Press.

Rogers CR (1952) Toward a theory of creativity. In Rogers CR (1961) *On Becoming a Person: A Therapist's View of Psychotherapy.* London: Constable & Company Ltd.

Rogers CR (1957) The necessary and sufficient conditions of therapeutic personality change. *Journal of Consulting Psychology,* 21(2): 95-103.

Rogers CR (1961) *On Becoming a Person: a Therapist's View of Psychotherapy.* London: Constable & Company.

Rogers N (2000) *The Creative Connection. Expressive Arts as Healing.* Ross-on Wye: PCCS Books.

Romanyshyn R (2006). The wounded researcher: levels of transference in the research process. In HARVEST: International Journal for Jungian Studies, 52, 1, 38-49

Rosemont F (ed) (1981) *Isadora Speaks: Isadora Duncan.* San Francisco: City Lights Books.

Ruud E (1995) Improvisation as a liminal experience. In Bereznak Kenny C (ed) (1995) *Listening, Playing, Creating: Essays on the Power of Sound.* Albany, NY: State University of New York Press.

Schmais C (1985) Healing processes in group dance therapy. *American Journal of Dance Therapy,* 8, 17-36.

Schmais C, White E (1986) Introduction to Dance Therapy. *American Journal of Dance Therapy*, 9, 23-30.

Shakespeare W (1968) *Hamlet Prince of Denmark*. London: Penguin Books.

Siegel DJ (1999) *Developing Mind: Toward a Neurobiology of Interpersonal Experience*. New York, NY: Guilford.

Sills C, Fish S, Lapworth P (1995) Gestalt Counselling. Bicester: Winslow.

Skeat WW (1978) *A Concise Etymological Dictionary of the English Language*. Oxford: Oxford University Press.

Smith L (2005) Embodying Womanhood; the Effects of Fertility Choices on Women, Explored Through the Imagery of Butoh. Unpublished BA dissertation, University of Chichester.

Stanton-Jones K (1992) *Dance Movement Therapy in Psychiatry*. London: Routledge.

Steinman L (1995) The Knowing Body: The Artist as Storyteller in Contemporary Performance. Berkeley: North Atlantic Books.

Stern DN (1985) *The Interpersonal World of the Infant. A View from Psychoanalysis and Developmental Psychology*. New York, NY: Basic Books Inc.
Storr A (1976) *The Dynamics of Creation*. London: Pelican.

Svankmajer J (1965) J.S. Bach: fantasy in G minor. In Svankmajer J (1994) *Transmutation of the Senses*. Prague: Central Europe Gallery and Publishing House.

Thorne B (2002) The Mystical Power of Person-Centred Therapy, Hope Beyond Despair. London: Whurr Publishers Ltd.

Trungpa C (1996) *Dharma Art*. Boston MA: Shambhala Publications.

Tuby M (1996) Jung and the symbol: resolution of conflicting opposites. In Pearson J (ed) (1996) *Discovering the Self through*

Drama and Movement: The Sesame Approach. London: Jessica Kingsley Publishers.

Tufnell M, Crickmay C (1990) *Body Space Image.* London: Virago Press.

Valle R. Mohs M (1998) Transpersonal awareness in phenomenological inquiry: philosophy, reflections, and recent research. In Braud W, Anderson R (eds) (1998) *Transpersonal Research Methods for the Social Sciences: Honoring Human Experience.* London: Sage.

Whitehouse M (1958a) The Tao of the body. Paper presented at the Analytical Psychology Club of Los Angeles. In Pallaro P (ed) (1999) *Authentic Movement : Essays by Mary Starks Whitehouse, Janet Adler and Joan Chodorow.* London: Jessica Kingsley Publishers.

Whitehouse M (1958b) Movement experience: the raw material of dance. *Contact Quarterly* (2002), Summer/ Fall.

Whitehouse M (1972) In Frantz G (ed) An approach to the center: an interview with Mary Whitehouse. *Psychological Perspectives*, 3, 1, 37-46.

Whitehouse M (1978) Conversation with Mary Whitehouse and Frieda Sherman. *American Journal of Dance Therapy*, 2 (2), 3-4.

Whitehouse M (1979) C.G. Jung and dance therapy. In Pallaro P (ed) (1999) *Authentic Movement: Essays by Mary Starks Whitehouse, Janet Adler and Joan Chodorow.* London: Jessica Kingsley Publishers.

Winnicott DW (1971) *Playing and Reality.* London: Tavistock Publications.

Winterson J (1996) *Art Objects : Essays on Ecstasy and Effrontery.* London: Vintage.

Woodman M (1982) *Addiction to Perfection: The Still Unravished Bride.* Toronto: Inner City Books.

Woodman M (1993) *Conscious Femininity*. Toronto: Inner City Books.

Wyatt G (ed) (2001) *Congruence*. Ross-on-Wye: PCCS Books.

Yalom ID (1991) *Love's Executioner and Other Tales of Psychotherapy*. Harmondsworth: Penguin.

WEBSITES

www.admt.org.uk

www.admt.org.uk/ emotion

www.AuthenticMovement-BodySoul.com

www.baat.org

www.catmclelland.com

www.creativevoicework.com

www.danzasensibile.net

www.mwoodmanfoundation.org

www.mythinglinks.org

www.mythosandlogos.com

www.nnah.org.uk

www.resurgence.org

www.stillness.co.uk

www.tamalpa.org

INDEX OF NAMES

Printed in the United Kingdom
by Lightning Source UK Ltd.
123174UK00001B/82-105/A